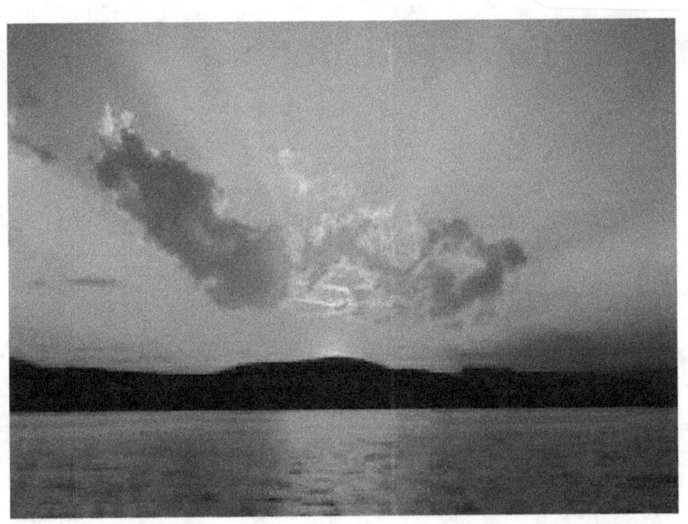

The Diabetes Handbook

A Solution to Diabetes
By Mary A. White

When the acidity is in the pancreas, diabetes is the result. (Pg 23)."

From the book, **The ph Miracle for Diabetes** by
Robert O. Young, MD

Table of Contents

Chapter One

Before We Begin:

Penicillin (our first antibiotic) was discovered in 1893. But it was not used until 1943, when the many medical emergencies of WWII caused it to be tried. So how was it that we were denied the use of this fantastic medicine for 50 years? How many people were in pain or died unnecessarily during those 50 years who could have been saved by antibiotics?

The answer to why it was not used for 50 years is that it took 50 years for the mainstream medical establishment to begin to believe that it worked. It took 50 years for this new knowledge to work itself through the medical system.

It is important to remember this story about penicillin as you read this booklet. For we believe that the information in this booklet is also 50 years ahead of its time. The mainstream medical establishment is just now beginning to ponder on the possibility that most degenerative diseases and many of the causes of aging are caused by acid deposits in the body. It doesn't even begin to state what may be causing these toxic deposits to form there.

We don't have 50 years to wait for their enlightenment. So plunge in, read this booklet and get 50 years (at least) ahead of the system.

Chapter Two:

Background and Overview

(Our Message In a Nutshell)

How I found a Diabetes Solution

When I was 62 years old I had arthritis. For 7 years my body had slowly stiffened up with arthritis. I had reached the point that I could not pick up anything that fell on the floor. That was a frustrating feeling. Plus, many normal recreational and hobby pursuits were no longer possible. Heck, I could not even put on my socks without pain.

I have an avid interest in holistic medicine and natural healing. So for years I have read everything that I could find about arthritis and associated diseases such as diabetes. I tried numerous remedies. My research on arthritis and the interactions of the human body that cause such affliction became an insatiable quest. I learned why arthritis and diabetes are more common today than ever before. Then I found the solution.

As with many great truths, the secret of how I cured my arthritis is very simple. And I learned that my arthritis solution is also the solution for some 150 other degenerative diseases, including diabetes. It will also be the solution for many of the other afflictions that are associated with aging. Once you read and understand my discovery, you will understand that it will probably resolve your diabetes problems. It also will help you to maintain your energy and overall vigor.

But first I have to explain some basic things about how your body works. Each individual cell of your body is an independent organism. It needs to be fed oxygen and food in order to live and prosper, and it also produces waste products that have to be removed from the cell for it to remain healthy. It is the job of your blood to perform these functions. Your blood carries fresh oxygen and food to each cell of your body, and then having completed this task, it picks up the waste products (also called toxins) from the cell. These waste products are carried by the blood to the walls of your intestines. There the waste products (toxins) are passed through the walls of the intestine, to be excreted from your body along with your body's food waste products.

That is how it is supposed to work, and that is how it works for most of us during our younger years. But as we age, things begin to change.

Your Body's *ph* Balance

Now let's talk about your body's acid/alkaline balance (also know as *ph*). Every farmer and agronomist will tell you that plants grow best in soils that have the proper *ph* for that plant. That is because every organism has a range of alkalinity/acidity in which it will prosper. Outside of that range of *ph,* the organism dies or is greatly stressed just to survive. Thus it is that corn will not grow well in soil that is too alkaline, and carrots will not grow well in soil that is too acidic.

Our bodies are the same. There is a range of acidity/alkalinity for our bodies in which they function perfectly. But should the body's acidity/alkalinity balance fall outside of this range, the body becomes stressed, its ability to function properly becomes decreased, and eventually this stressed condition will lead to a degenerative disease that may eventually cause death.

In today's world, there is a strong tendency for our bodies to become too acidic. That is because we eat too much acidic food. Red meats are highly acidic, as is soda pop, most processed food, and fried foods. Even carbohydrates and sugars turn acidic during the digestion process. How many years has it been since my high school physics teacher soaked a dried chicken leg bone in a glass of coca cola? Within an hour the bone could be tied into a knot because of the acidity of the cola. But we tend to ignore all this. Thus it is that our bodies slowly tend to become acidic. It is a slow process, and we don't notice it. That is okay when we are in our twenties and thirties. But by the time we reach our forties, fifties and sixties, the accumulated effect of eating too much acidic food begins to show up as pain, and our bodies become dangerously acidic.

Lets talk specifics here. At a *ph* of 7.2, the body is in perfect *ph* balance, neither too acidic or too alkaline. A *ph* range of 7.0 to 7.5 is the acceptable range for a body to be in good health. When the *ph* drops to between 6.5 and 7.0, the body is beginning to get stressed and fatigue and a feeling of pain or lethargy begins to set in. When the *ph* drops to between 6.0 and 6.5, the body is beginning to become seriously acidic, and it is probably developing one or more of the 150 specific degenerative diseases or pains that are associated with an acetic condition. Then when your *ph* gets to between 6.0 and 5.5, you are in serious trouble, your energy levels are shot, and a degenerative disease or pain of some sort is upon you.

When I discovered this very simple but crucial bit of information, I checked my *ph*. It was 5.5. No wonder I was having health problems!

Chapter Three

How Degenerative Disease (Including Diabetes) Begins

Now lets talk about how this situation leads to degenerative diseases such as arthritis, diabetes and cancer. Okay, you have led a good life, used moderation in most things, and have good health. But gradually, unknown to you, your body acidity has slowly, over the years, increased. As your acidity has increased, your body has experienced several reactions to this changed condition. A general feeling of fatigue and tiredness has set in. But also, the acidic condition of your blood now affects its ability to perform a function that it used to perform with ease. The ability of your stressed blood to carry food and oxygen to the body's cells, and its ability to carry away the waste products from the cells is lessened.

Your blood, now unable to easily perform these functions, becomes overloaded with waste products (toxins) that it cannot easily dispose of. So it looks for other ways to dispose of the waste products. Some of them it stores in your fat deposits. Others it stores as deposits in the linings of your veins and arteries, or in your pancreas. And others it deposits on places where your bones are exposed, such as the bone joints of your body. It is these deposits of certain toxins (waste products) in your bone joints that eventually manifest as arthritis. **The deposits of toxins that accumulate in your pancreas will cause diabetes.**

So, as I have outlined here, my arthritis was in actuality caused by a long-term over-acidity in my body. Once I realized this, I began to look for a direct and simple treatment to change my *ph* balance (acidy/alkalinity) back to a healthy range. Eventually I found a blend of mineral compounds and herbs that gave me pain relief, leading to total symptom reversal.

After I began treatment, my recovery from arthritis was dramatic. Within 6 weeks of treatment my *ph* had gone from 5.5 to 6.5. Not only did my arthritis stiffness and symptoms begin to disappear, I also regained much of my prior energy and zest for life. Now my acidity levels are in the healthy range, and it is easy for me to keep them that way. What I especially like is that no draconian diet changes were necessary.

Chapter Four:

The Problem With Dieting

There have been many shifts in healing beliefs in the last twenty years. One of these shifts is the gradual but persistent growth in the understanding that diet and nutrition are vitally important in maintaining good health and conquering many illnesses. Now, if you peruse the available information on natural or alternative medicine approaches and therapies, you will be bombarded with a plethora of guidance about proper foods to eat, recommended diets, etc.

Likewise, when many holistic-oriented experts counsel you about your illness, they will point out the acidity-disease connection. They will recommend/suggest what is usually a very rigid and strict diet. Basically, they will tell you not to eat acidic foods (red meat) and to only eat vegetables and fruits (alkaline foods). The idea is that an all-alkaline diet will cause the acidity in your body to lessen enough for the conditions in your body that caused the disease conditions to reverse themselves, thus reducing the symptoms of the disease. What they will suggest to you is a diet approach such as the following:

Alkalizing With Food

Your diet should consist of an 80/20 balance: eighty percent of your food should be an alkaline food, and 20% of your food should be an acidic food. This balance will eventually affect your acid/alkaline balance, raising your ph to an acceptable level.

A List of Alkaline Foods is as follows:

Vegetables*:* asparagus, watercress, fermented vegetables(sauerkraut, **etc.**), beets, broccoli, Brussels sprouts, cabbage, carrots, cauliflower, celery, chard, collard greens, cucumber, eggplant, garlic, kale, kohlrabi, lettuce, mushrooms, mustard, onions, parsnips, peas, peppers, pumpkin, spirulina, sprouts, squash, alfalfa, wild greens and nightshade vegetables.

Fruits: apple, apricot, avocado, banana, cantaloupe, cherries, dates, figs, grapes, grapefruit, lime, honeydew melon, oranges, lemon, peach, pear, pineapple, berries, tomato, watermelon, and all tropical fruits.

Protein: almonds, chestnuts, chicken, cottage cheese, eggs, nuts, pumpkin seeds, sunflower seeds, tofu, and yogurt.

A List of the Acidic Foods that you must avoid is:

Protein: beef, fish, clams, shellfish, crustaceans (lobster and shrimp), turkey, and venison.

Fats and Oils: All salad and cooking oils, olive oil, and lard.

Grains: All breakfast cereal grains (wheat, barley, corn), oats, rice, and rye. All breads.

Nuts and Butters: All nuts and peanut butter.

Beans and Legumes: All beans, peas and soy.

Dairy: Cheese, milk and butter.

Bev*erages:* Beer, distilled water, liquor, and wine.

Fruit and Vegetables: Blueberries, glazed or canned fruits, cranberries, plums, prunes, corn, olives, potatoes, and winter squash.

Are They Crazy or What?

If you are like me, when you reviewed this above list of forbidden foods (acidic foods), you thought to yourself,

"I would rather be dead than follow this diet!". No beef, no bread, no potatoes, no seafood, no cheese? Yes, the above type of alkalizing diet is too stringent for most of us. So what else can we do? Well that is the purpose of this booklet; to explain to you a much simpler way to reduce the acid levels in your body down to a healthy level so that your diabetes goes away.

Chapter Five

More About Acids in Your Body

The concept that an acid/alkaline imbalance in the body is a major cause of disease isn't new. Remember Edgar Cayce, the famous sleeping prophet from back in the 1930s and 1940s? He often suggested body detoxification, colonics, fasting, massage, steam baths and alkalizing the body by diet modification (see our addendum). He also on occasion recommended ingesting baking soda as a remedy for overacidity and diabetes.

Back in 1933 Dr. William Howard published a breakthrough book titled *A New Health Era* in which he postulated that self-poisoning by acid accumulation in the body was a major cause of all illnesses. He stated, "We depart from health in the proportion to which we have allowed our alkalis to be dissipated by the introduction of too much acid forming food. It may seem strange to say, but all disease is the same thing, no matter what its form of expression, but it is so."

As we presently live, very few of us can rid our bodies of all the acids that we create from stress, foods, and our metabolisms. These acid wastes move around the body via the blood and lymphatic system until they reach our kidneys. Our kidneys are many times overloaded with toxin accumulation, so that they cannot process the new waste. Our blood and lymphatic fluid, unable to dispose of the acid waste in the kidneys, seeks an alternative way to get rid of the waste. They must do this so that they can resume their main job of carrying oxygen and nutrients t the cells of the body. So the blood and lymphatic fluid take an alternate route; they dispose of the acid waste by dumping it into our fat, veins, organs, or bone joints (the resulting deposits thus causing arthritis) or the pancreas (resulting in diabetes). Both cholesterol and crystallized uric acid are formed from the "dumped" acid wastes that could not be processed by the kidneys.

Harmful Effects of Acid

Acid coagulates blood. Also blood has problems flowing around fatty acids, and thus tends to clump. Capillaries then clog up and die. The skin, deprived of life-giving blood, loses elasticity and begins to wrinkle. We begin to look old.

It is not only your skin. Without a proper acid/alkaline balance, every part of the body works harder to maintain health. All systems (lungs, organs, skin, etc.) work to and depend on the maintenance of a correct blood pH. Your organs and cells are totally subservient to your blood and the blood acid level (pH). All organs work to keep your blood at a balanced pH, to the point where your body is willing to inflict major damages on other parts of your body that stand in the way of a correct blood pH. In other words, your body will damage itself in order to keep a proper blood pH. This is because if the blood pH strays out of a very narrow range, you will die.

The Proper PH Level:

If your blood pH dips from its optimal pH of 7.2 down to lower levels (becomes acidic) your health will suffer. The proper blood pH is very critical! So your body knows what it doing when it disposes of acid wastes in various locations within your body. These accumulations of acidic wastes eventually cause you disease and pain. Better disease than death.

One of the reasons that you get a charge from drinking a cola (pH of 2.5, very acidic) is that this acidity sets off alarm bells all over your body. The resulting surge of adrenaline gives you the rush that you get from the cola. Alkaline chemicals that are stored in your body rush to neutralize the acids. This deprives the rest of your body of these alkalizing chemicals (such as calcium in your bones).

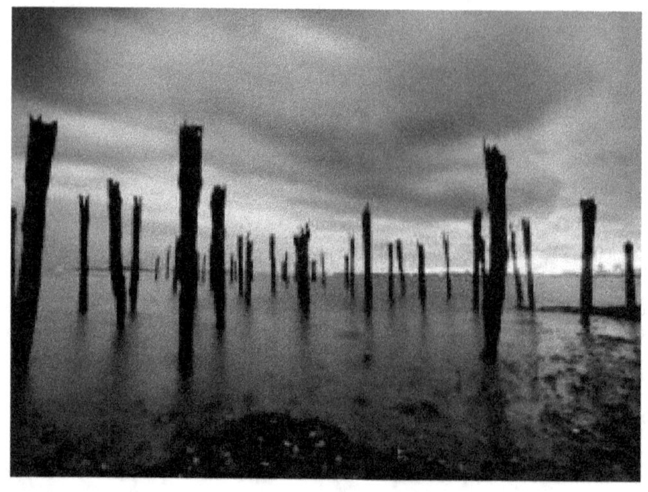

The "high" that you got from drinking that cola is no different from the "high" a drug user gets as he experiences his artificial sensory elevation. The high is your body screaming for help, and not knowing the difference, you enjoy the feeling. It is not just the cola that causes such effect. Most of us already have a running battle within our body as our body struggles to deal with and counteract the effects of too much acid-causing foods, and acid-causing stress in our system.

About Stress: Of all the acidifying factors, stress is the greatest. Stress can neutralize and acidify an alkaline diet with just one surge of adrenaline. This is important. We can show you how to reduce the acid levels in your body to a healthy level, but you must also work hard to keep the stress low in your life. If there is unavoidable stress, learn to control it or to channel it so that its effect on you is minimized.

Long Term Effects of Acidity

We have 60,000 miles of veins and arteries in our bodies. Acids eat into and corrode these veins and arteries. If left unchecked, it eventually interrupts or damages all cellular activity and function, to even include the beating of our heart to the nerve functions within our brain.

In addition, if the blood cells are so loaded with toxins that they cannot dispose of, the blood cells cannot carry enough oxygen back to the body cells to meet their oxygen needs. Thus the body's cells get starved for oxygen. This is really catastrophic. Without sufficient oxygen, the cells get stressed, then weaken, then age prematurely, then die.

Incredibly, Dr. Otto Warburg in 1934 was awarded the Nobel Prize for discovering that cancer was caused by a lack of oxygen in the body cells. He found that when the oxygen level of your blood falls below 60 percent of normal, an anaerobic condition is created in which cancer can prosper [anaerobic means "absence of oxygen"]. It actually is quite simple. The cancer virus is anaerobic; that is, it can only live in an absence of oxygen. Cancer cells exposed to oxygen will die. An obvious solution for cancer, and many other illnesses (including AIDS) is to maintain oxygen levels in the body above the 60 percent level.

Why the mainstream medical establishment has ignored these facts for some seventy years is interesting. I will leave it to you to ponder on this.

In summary, over-acidity damages life itself, leading to all forms of sickness and disease, as well as general symptoms of aging. As you are probably beginning to realize, this story is just not about a certain disease and how to cure it, it is also about explaining to you one of the principal causes of disease and aging, and telling you how to correct the matter. This is powerful stuff. If you are like me, you will eventually be thankful for this knowledge. You will appreciate this for having opened up your knowledge and awareness so that you can maintain a much healthier body and lead a much longer and healthier life. **Without good health, we have nothing!**

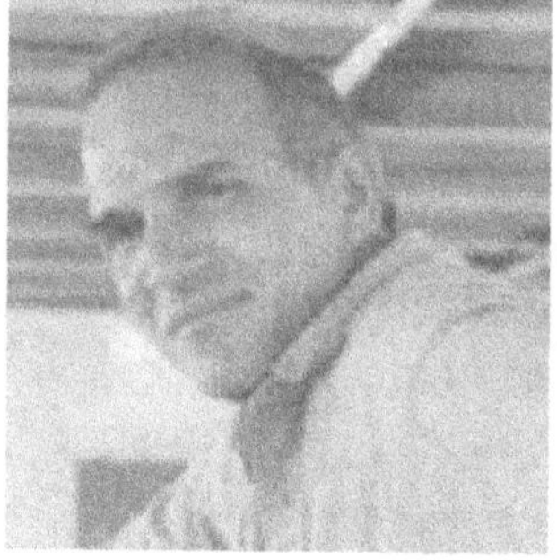

In his book, *Alkalize or Die*, Dr. Theodore A. Baroody, MD states, "Too much acidity in the body is like having too little oil in the car. It just grinds to a halt one day and dies. There you are-stuck. The body also does the same thing. It starts painfully creaking to a stop along the byways of life and you find yourself in some

kind of discomfort. I watch
with great concern as people of
all classes and lifestyles suffer
from this excess."

He attributes 68 major health conditions (including
diabetes, of course) to acidic conditions in the body. His
book is great to read, and I highly recommend it.

Chapter Six

All About Alkalinity and Blood

Your blood is meant to always be slightly alkaline. It must be slightly alkaline in order to maintain resistance to decay and the possible growth of bad or harmful organisms that can grow in an acidic environment. Therefore the blood has a very narrow range of pH in which it can operate. As we have previously (somewhat dramatically, for effect!) stated, if your blood gets outside of this acceptable range of pH, you will die.

The absolutely perfect pH level of your blood is 7.365. The pH level is that exact.

If the blood gets slightly outside this pH level, results will be felt in every part of your body. Harmful and poisoning organisms that can grow and multiply in an acidic environment begin to do so. They take on the function of aggressive, parasitic and pathogenic agents (a hint here for candida suffers of why you have a yeast infection in your body that does not go away).

Scientists and researchers can use a dark field microscope to see the changes in the blood that take place as blood acidity increases. They watch the repetitive pattern unfolding as disease organisms proliferate and grow, and they document the ensuing debilitation of the body that, if left unchecked, will eventually kill us, one way or another.

The Power of pH

The pH scale is logarithmic. This means that each pH value is ten times higher than the previous number. For example, if your pH goes from 7 to 6, it means that your body is **ten times** more acidic. This is very important to understand as you begin to monitor your blood acidity levels.

Your goal should be to maintain a body pH level of somewhere around 7. I am able to eat whatever I want and still maintain a pH level of from 6.6 to 7.0 by using the practices that this book will explain. This keeps me happy, I feel great, and I live with the knowledge that many diseases, such as cancer, etc, will have a hard time living in my body. All this, in addition to the fact that my arthritis has gone away!

A glass of cola has a pH of 2.5 (very acidic). It is approximately 50,000 times more acidic than a glass of water! One of the active ingredients in cola is phosphoric acid. Not to beat up too much on colas, but when I was in a high school science class (a long time ago), my teacher conducted an experiment. He placed a dried-out chicken drumstick bone in a container of cola. After only 30 minutes he removed the previously dried out and rigid chicken leg bone from the cola, and he then tied it into a knot. The cola had softened the bone that much! All this to demonstrate to us the acidity of colas. I guess

that I wasn't too impressed, because I kept right on
drinking colas until just a few years ago when my
arthritis caused me to wise up in this matter. Now I drink
bottled diet iced tea from the vending machines.

I consider a body pH level of 7.0 to be good. Conversely,
if your blood pH level dropped to 7.0 you would die. It
would mean that your blood (with an ideal level of ph
7.365) had become almost four times too acidic. You
would then die from blood poisoning. All this is to
explain to you that the rest of your body is totally
committed to maintaining your blood at the correct pH,
and the rest of your body will sacrifice itself totally
(including giving itself disease) in order to protect the
pH level of your blood.

I hope that I have explained this satisfactorily. Whereas
your body can and does function at a wide range of pH
(basically from 7.2 to 5.5), your blood does not. Your
body knows this, and does everything possible to protect
the blood pH. This protection includes sacrificing other
body functions and parts in order to protect the blood. So
your disease is part of your body's efforts to protect the
pH level of your blood. Your body, believe it or not,
knew what it was doing when it gave you an illness or
made you fat!

The Alkalinity and Parasite Connection

As we have explained, acidity in your body permits disease organisms to grow and thrive. This includes simple germs, yeasts, fungi, viruses and molds. These microorganisms all produce excretions (excrement). These excretions are toxic to your body. The organisms not only eat glucose, fats and protein from our bodies, they also poison our bodies with the resulting excretions. In short, they take our food and turn it into poison.

Again, the symptoms of this parasite poisoning may not be patently obvious, but they are there. They manifest as the gradual weakening of our bodies that we otherwise attribute to aging, tiredness, overwork, etc.

It is kind of like when a lumberjack cuts down a big tree with his axe. It takes many whacks from the axe before the tree falls, each small whack removing a tiny portion of the tree. But the tree does eventually fall, the cumulative effects of the many small whacks taking their effect. Well, consider the parasite poisoning in your body as one of those small whacks. Watch out, or eventually you will also, as did the big tree, fall and die. Get rid of those parasites now by balancing the pH levels in your body. Get rid of your acidity!

Alkalinity and Minerals

As you know, minerals are essential to your health. Properly assimilating the minerals into your body is also important. Many of you have read how much of the nutritive value of the mineral supplements that we take is lost to us because our bodies do not properly assimilate the minerals in their supplement form.

Each mineral has its own special "signature" pH level that it needs in order to be assimilated into your body. This is critical to understand. I repeat: each mineral has its own special "signature" pH level that it needs in order to be assimilated into your body.

Every chemistry classroom has a chart of periodic elements, including all minerals. Those minerals at the lower end are capable of being assimilated in the body over a broader range of body pH. Those higher on the chart require a much narrower range of pH in order to be assimilated. In short, if your body is too acidic your body will simply reject many minerals that are critical to your health.

One example of why this is important: Look at iodine. It is high on the periodic scale, and therefore requires almost perfect pH levels in the body in order to be assimilated. Iodine is required for a healthy thyroid. If our body is too acidic, the thyroid will receive insufficient iodine, and thus cannot perform properly. A malfunctioning thyroid is connected to arthritis, cancer, diabetes, heart attacks depression, fatigue and obesity.

Yet few of us are able to connect the dots and recognize that these illnesses are caused by your malfunctioning thyroid, which is caused by overacidity. Interesting, is it not? Tragic, is it not?

This mineral assimilation situation is made worse because our agricultural lands have become mineral depleted. Overuse of chemical fertilizers (that only provide three of the eight-two necessary minerals and trace elements that our bodies need) and overuse of insecticides and pesticides have caused our soils to not provide our fruits and vegetables with the minerals that we need. It has been shown that today's vegetables only provide 25% of the mineral nutrition that they provided 70 years ago (before the introduction of chemical fertilizers after WWII.). This in itself is an interesting story, too long to tell here. But it bears merit for further study on your part. Lets fix your diabetes first!

Dr. William R. Kellas, MD is author of the book *Surviving in a Toxic World.* He says that your pH level plays an important part in ridding your body of mercury and other harmful metals. Heavy metals such as mercury harm your body through oxidative stress that in turn leads to higher acidity

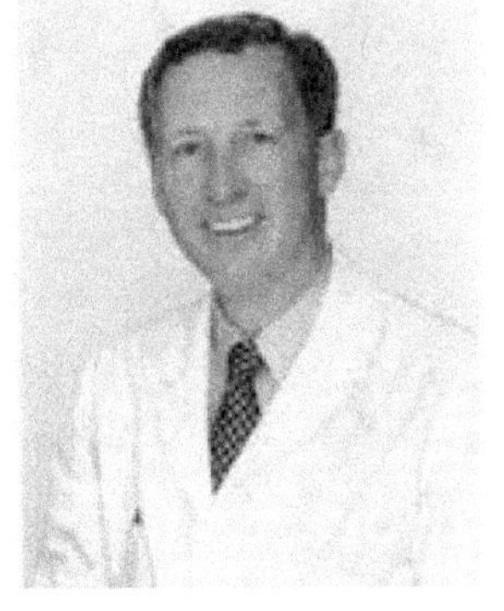

Alzheimer's disease, among others, is believed caused by

mercury poisoning in the body.
Dr. Kellas provides pH test strips
to his patients so they can
measure and track their pH as
they detoxify. We will explain
how you can do this later in the
book.

As you begin to de-acidify your body, you may
experience a variety of detoxification symptoms such as
headaches, body pains and aches, stiffness, itching, etc.
These signs are often referred to as a "healing crisis" and
they are your body's way of telling you that it is being
changed (for the better).

Chapter Seven

Is Your Fat Saving Your Life?

Many of us suffer the pains and arrows of outrageous fortune due to obesity. Yes. Fat is a major problem in today's world. But it is not just that we eat too much or that we eat the wrong foods. Believe it or not, overacidity in our bodies also causes us to be fat. This explains why many of us (myself included) do not respond satisfactorily to diet and exercise. We fast and work out, and the fat still doesn't come off. What gives?

Our bodies actually resist giving up the fat because the fat is actually saving our lives. Is this a wild statement or what?

Why Our Bodies Cling To Their Fat

Dr. Lynda Frassetto, MD, from the University of California has researched this matter. She believes that humans, in evolutionary terms, have changed. Once upon a time, our bodies used to break down food and dispose of the acid waste with our kidneys and livers. But now, because of the sheer amount of acid waste the average American produces, she sees our inner bodies being turned into a war zone, where our body is fighting

to protect its most strategic reserves --- our kidney and
liver -- from total degradation and failure.

One of the ways that our body does this is by finding
somewhere else to store the body waste products
(including crystallized uric acid). May times this
somewhere else is the fatty deposits. So, as far as your
body is concerned, you fat is important to it because it
has your waste toxins stored there.

You exercise and diet in order to make your fat go away.
But your body says to itself, "I need that Fat. That is my
warehouse for stored toxins." So it holds onto the fat. It
resists losing weight. And you get frustrated because you
remain fat because you do not understand the real
problem. The real problem is overacidity in your body.
We seem a bit redundant here, don't we? But it is
important for you to appreciate this wisdom and
knowledge. In actuality, your body thinks that it is
saving your life by clinging onto that fat!

An Evolutionary Change

(Author's Note) Some of this info provided by Dr.
Frassetto below repeats information that we have already
covered. But a bit of redundancy here may be in order,
as this information is so darn important!

To prove this theory, Dr. Frassetto studied 1000 people
and discovered that we are indeed stockpiling acid waste
in our fatty deposits instead of eliminating it with our
kidneys and liver. Cholesterol and crystallized uric acid

are solidified acids that have been dumped within the body for later disposal, which never comes. Our bodies have made the choice to preserve our kidney and liver instead of processing the acid waste. The cost is tremendous -- obesity, low energy, and many acid related diseases such as osteoarthritis, diabetes, cancer, painful periods, and much more.

When our bodies are excessively acidic, they borrow essential minerals such as calcium, sodium, potassium, and magnesium from our vital organs and bones to buffer or neutralize the acid. The result is our bodies suffer from prolonged degradation or corrosion, which manifests into these dehabilitating conditions and pains.

The reason is simple -- the average American diet contains way too much acid. Diet coke and other soda is probably the most acidic food people consume at a pH of 2.5. Beer and meat are at 3.5, then there's dairy, white pasta, most water, wine, hard alcohol, nuts and butters, beans, oils -- all acidic foods. All produce acid waste in our bodies that they can't handle. Dr. Robert O. Young agrees with Dr. Frassetto's theory. Sugar is an acid and she sees Westerners consumption of sugar as the reason why so many are overweight. The body has to protect itself from the excess sugar, so it creates fat to encase the acid. "Fat," she says. "Is saving our lives."
Then there's the problem of disease. The stomach works by producing acid to break down food. Whenever this acid is made, alkaline buffers are also created and sent through our blood stream, naturally alkalizing our body. A healthy balanced body has alkaline reserves to battle

diseases, infections, and viruses. But if excessive acid must be continuously neutralized or stored, our alkaline reserves will be depleted, leaving our bodies weakened and disease prone.

Acid and Stress

Dr. Frassetto says that acid comes from three sources -- food, pollution, and stress. Of these three, stress is the greatest problem. One shot of adrenaline can neutralize and acidify an alkaline diet. So stress management as well as diet management is essential to maintaining an alkaline body that is free of pain.

She says that the worst case scenario in which many Westerners fit into is where we work 40-50 hour stressful weeks with hardly any breaks to calm ourselves down. We consume fast food and coffee for quick bursts of artificial energy to just get through our workday. Then we come home to family stresses, household chores, bills, and more and never really relax and give our bodies a chance to neutralize all the acid we produced through stress and from eating very acidic foods. So acid in our bodies build up until we begin to show symptoms -- digestive problems, headaches, overweight, bone pains, elimination issues, muscle tension and pain, heart problems, high blood pressure, and more. We spend our lives giving ourselves to our jobs and families and never take the time to nourish our bodies, mind, and soul.

More Effects of Acid on our Body

Dr. Frassetto also says that acidity is like rust. Our veins and arteries are corroded by acid. If nothing is done, acid interrupts all cellular activities and functions -- from our beating heart to the way we think. Blood also can't flow around fatty acids so capillaries clog up and die. Our skin begins to wrinkle and isn't as stretchy. Pains develop. Even if you put out the money for a face-lift or liposuction, the acid still remains and will do damage. As for our lungs and other organs, all are involved in the maintenance of correct blood pH so if all have to work harder to deal with excessive acid, all will stop functioning a whole lot sooner than we want them to. Did you know that if any substance changes from a 7 to an 8 pH, it has become ten times more alkaline? The opposite is also true, if it changes from a 7 pH to a 6, it has become ten times more acidic.

Chapter Eight

Lets Talk About Our Solution

My Epiphany

Well, I have previously explained that arthritis pain had begun to cripple me. My aching knees were keeping me awake at night. My doctor suggested knee replacement surgery (ouch!). This forced me out of desperation to begin my own research on arthritis. I had previously beaten cancer by discovering my own alternative remedy (Essiac Herbal Tea), so I was determined to do the same thing for my arthritis pain.

Could this be it? So simple! Our bodies have too much acid. If I ingest a base (baking soda, also known as sodium bicarbonate, jumped to mind) would it react with some of the acid in my body to make a salt, a salt that my body could easily expel? Wow. What an interesting idea. So I began daily eating about 8,000 mg (a small teaspoonful) of Arm and Hammer Baking Soda. I bought it at the grocery store. I mixed it with water. It tasted yucky. Within a month I began to see results. Within three months I began to regain my flexibility. All pain was gone. Later I had a chemist put the baking soda in capsules. That tasted much better. No more yucky taste.

So now, even though my arthritis has gone bye-bye, I still take my capsules daily. I test my pH weekly, keeping it always above 6.6 or 6.7. Usually it tests out at about 7.0. And I feel twenty years younger.

Further research led me to understand that there are cell salts that also correct diabetes and arthritis. So I added this to my formulas, along with some special herbs that also are remedies for diabetes and arthritis. I shared my information freely. Others have marketed my formulas in capsule form. For further information about how to obtain the diabetes product, go to www.nhe.net/diabetestype12treatment. The arthritis product can be found at the website www.nhe.net/arthritistreatment.

How Will You Know That It Is Working?

I previously mentioned that there are test strips that you can use to test your body's pH. Remember litmus paper in high school chemistry? It is very similar.

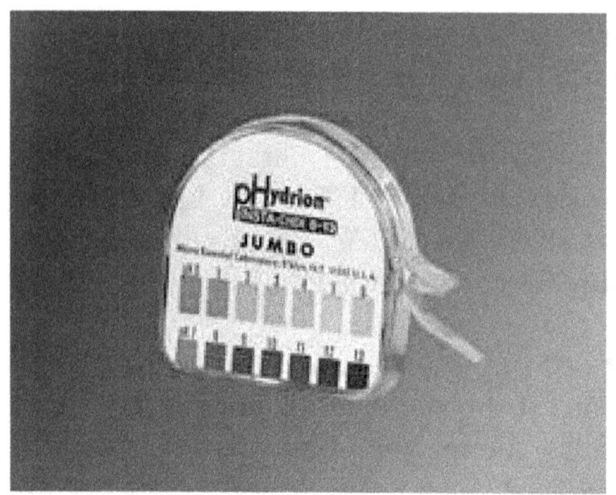

Shown is a typical test kit that you can buy. I buy mine off the Internet. The test kit shown is found on www.microessentiallab.com.

It is Catalog # 067, Hydrion Single Roll pH Paper and sells for $7.50.

I test my saliva in the morning before I have brushed my teeth or eaten anything.

How To Test For Your pH

Saliva pH is controlled by your diet and the amount of
vitamins and minerals you have in your body. Lower
saliva pH is a good indicator that the body is too acidic.
Saliva pH over 7.0 is a good indicator that you are in
excellent health.. This simple test is a good general way
to measure the level of your acidity. The benefits of
saliva pH testing are that it is simple, inexpensive, and
the patient has control over monitoring their path back to
good health. Saliva pH has been used by physicians for
decades as a general indicator of your body's health, as
well as the specific check we seek for treatment of
diabetes or arthritis.

Recent research has linked low saliva pH to numerous
leading diseases, including diabetes. Saliva pH is usually
measured from 5-9, the lower your score the more acidic
and the more likely you are to have health problems.
Your ideal saliva pH level should be between 7.0-7.4,
this is either 1st thing in the morning or an hour after any
food or fluid intake. The good news is that you can
monitor and improve your health without costly
medications or doctors visits. You can improve your
saliva pH by improving the foods you eat and the
nutritional supplements you take. Then you can say
goodbye to diabetes symptoms.

Quotes From Knowledgeable Doctors:

The below information is extracted from the wonderful and informative books about pH balance written by Dr. Robert O. Young, Microbiologist:

Forward in one book is by Chi C. Mao, M.D., Ph. D., Chief Medical Officer, Select Specialty Hospitals of Houston, Texas, a scientist who served previously at the National Institute of Health. He states:

1. According to mainstream medicine, arthritis and diabetes mellitus (either type 1 or type 2) have long been considered incurable.
2. Dr. Robert O. Young presents medical research, including clinical studies that suggest that a complete cure is possible.
3. Dr. Young's message is that "overacidification of our body fluids, due to our diet and modern lifestyles, is the origin of myriad pain and illnesses; therefore, in order to regain our health, it becomes imperative to minimize acidification and restore a critical balance."
4. Dr. Mao states, "It is my belief that Dr. Young's theory, his therapeutic methodology, and his commitment to health care will continue to make history in years to come."

"[Disease] results, rather, from a disruption of the delicate pH balance (acid-base) in the fluids that surround the cells of the pancreas and other organs. Overacidity in the fluid allows cells to transform in negative ways, interfering with (among many other things) the way the body produces and uses its energy, and causing pain.

"[Disease] is the result of a pH imbalance in the fluids of the body –systemic acidosis- that interferes with the optimum functioning of the cells they surround. Beta cells surrounded by acids do not or cannot produce sufficient insulin. Acids destroy insulin receptor sites on the cellular membrane so body cells cannot properly use the hormone."

"The one indicator most crucial to your health [is] the pH of your blood"

"Acidity in different tissues of the body shows up with different sets of symptoms and pain, which have had various labels slapped on them by mainstream medical science. When the acidity is in the pancreas, diabetes is the result."

> "In addition, when the blood is overly acid, it begins to unload the excess acids into the body's tissues, storing them in protective fat in the breasts, hips, belly, and even in the brain, heart, and pancreas."

"It would seem that our fat is killing us. And far be it from me to argue for carrying around excess baggage. But the truth is, right now all that fat is probably *saving* your life. That's because the body uses fat to bind up and neutralize its excess acids, protecting all the tissues and organs that sustain life from acid damage."

How to ingest Baking Soda

Many people take baking soda as a health assist by mixing baking soda in water and drinking it. Baking soda mixed with water tastes yucky. So I have found a way to take my baking soda that is more pleasant.

1. Start off taking about a quarter of a teaspoon once or twice daily. Work up from this until you are taking ¾ to a full teaspoonful once or twice daily.
2. Place your dosage of baking soda in a large empty glass. Add an equal amount of Tang or sweetened Kool-Aid. I also add powdered Splenda as a sweetener.

3. Fill the glass one-quarter full of water. Let whatever frothing occurs happen.
4. After the frothing has stopped, fill the glass the rest of the way with more water. Then stir thoroughly and drink.

I also mix some psyllium husk powder into my drink. Psyllium husks swell when they get to your stomach. This will give your stomach a full feeling, thus making dieting easier. And the psyllium husks also does a good job of cleaning your large intestine (colon). You can find bulk psyllium at many health food stores or order it off the Internet at sources such as herbalcom.com.

Additional Notes on taking Baking Soda

The big problem with taking baking soda is the terrible taste. I have worked out a method for taking it that works for me and I would like to share it with you. Every day I make a jar of sun (solar) tea. Two or three times a day I do the following: I take an 8 oz. glass of the tea, add stevia to taste, and then add 1/3 heaping teaspoon of baking soda. I stir thoroughly, and enjoy the drink. It is actually enjoyable after a while. I sometimes add a small amount of orange juice or other juice to vary the taste. I am sure to add enough stevia to make the taste pleasant.

When an opened box of baking soda is kept in the pantry it absorbs bad odors. These odors accumulate in the baking soda, adding to its unpleasant taste. So when I open a fresh box of baking soda, I place it in a small glass jar so I can keep it sealed to keep bad tastes away from it. This makes a big difference in how the baking soda drink tastes.

Another helpful tip that will improve the taste of your baking soda: Only use plastic spoons or other utensils to handle your baking soda. The baking soda will actually pick up an unpleasant metallic taste from a metal spoon or scoop. So only use plastic. I was amazed at how the taste of my baking soda drink improved with this simple trick.

My goal is to keep my body ph above 6.2. I believe that cancer cannot exist in your body at this ph. It also will help the other afflictions stay away. I am enclosing several ebooks on this subject. I am indebted to Dr. R.O. Young and his research on the connection between body ph and disease.

Diabetes is a big problem these days. It is caused by over-acidity of the pancreas. So the baking soda will help but it may take time. Arthritis sufferers can see dramatic results within a month. Cancer people can see results within several months.

Big business has taken over aspects of our life. There is no money to be made with baking soda health therapies, so you will never hear much about it from the system. Sorry, but that is just the way it is.

Chapter Nine

Conclusion

I hope that I have shown you how to prevent disease, keep your skin and organs healthy, and how to alkalize your body so that the body's natural systems will dispose of your unwanted body fat. It is so simple. Eat baking soda in an amount sufficient to remove the acidity from your body.

We read in our history books how the ancient Romans poisoned themselves by cooking in lead pots. Some historians even suggest that the resulting widespread lead poisoning of the general populace may have hastened the downfall of the Roman Empire.

We now know better than to eat in lead pots.

But could it just be that our own civilization is at a point where it is doing something equally stupid and disastrous? Could it be that many years from now students will read that our civilization weakened and perished because we over-acidified our bodies to the point that we poisoned ourselves and weakened our society? I have only to go to a shopping center and look at the shoppers. The general obesity and look of unhealthiness of our general populace is alarming.

I sincerely hope and pray that this small book will make a difference.

Attached is a copy of the informative and helpful book *Alternative Medicine Cancer Therapies.*

Addendum To Diabetes Health Book:

Edgar Cayce Information On Acidity

Some of this information is taken from the Meridian Institute Website .www.meridianinstitute.com

This background data is provided to assist you to understand the pain relief that is available for diabetes, arthritis, and other diseases, pain relief, and their symptoms.

ACID/ALKALINE BALANCE

Edgar Cayce consistently emphasized the importance of maintaining a proper acid/alkaline balance in the body. Commonly referred to as "pH" (potential for hydrogen), the acid/alkaline continuum ranges from 0 - 14 with 7 as neutral. The lower end of the scale (below 7) is acid and above 7 is alkaline. Generally speaking, the Cayce readings maintain that a balanced pH with a slight alkaline tendency would be beneficial for most individuals.

Edgar Cayce noted that high systemic acidity either causes or contributes to many health problems. The items on Scale 5 are based on 133 readings which mention "superacidity" as an etiological factor. High systemic acidity (Scale 5) is often caused by eating a diet containing too much acid producing foods such as sweets and meats. Stress is another factor which can increase acidity. Improper food combinations (such as eating grains and citrus at the same meal) can result in high acidity.

Alkalinity can be increased by consuming less meat and sweets and more vegetables and fruits. Although eating fruit to increase alkalinity may seem to be a contradiction because some fruits (especially citrus) are acidic outside the body, digestion uses up their acidic components, leaving an alkaline residue (ash). Thus the net effect is alkaline-producing within the system. For most individuals, Cayce noted that "a normal diet is about twenty percent acid to eighty percent alkaline-producing." Appendix F contains an acid/alkaline table that lists the Ph of common foods.

According to Cayce, numerous factors can increase acidity (and pain) including negative emotional states, inadequate mastication of food, and poor eliminations. Perhaps the most common factor cited by Cayce is diet. Eating acid-producing foods or combining foods improperly (even akaline-producing foods) is said to lead to hyperacidity, even to "superacidity" in some instances.

Cayce sometimes observed that infectious agents (such as virus and bacteria) do not thrive in an alkaline environment: "cold CANNOT - DOES NOT - exist in alkalines." Thus, consuming alkaline-producing foods (such as orange juice and lemon juice) was recommended to prevent colds.

The antimicrobial influence of alkalinity is supported by research on goldenseal, a well-known antibacterial herb. Berberine sulfate, the most active antibacterial alkaloid in goldenseal, is more effective in an alkaline than an acid environment. At a pH of 8.0 (alkaline), its antimicrobial activity in vitro is about 2 to 4 times greater than at 7.0 (neutral). At an acid pH of 6.0, the antimicrobial activity is only 1/4 as strong as at a neutral pH.

Acid/alkaline balance is extremely important to normal physiology. For example, the blood will maintain a slightly alkaline range of 7.35 to 7.45. Extended pH imbalances of any kind are not well tolerated by the body. The management of the pH factor is so important that the body has developed strict accounting procedures to monitor acid-alkaline balances in every cell and system. The fundamental regulatory systems of the body (including breathing, circulation, elimination, etc.) affect pH balance.

Edgar Cayce insisted that acid/alkaline balance could be easily checked. Numerous readings encourage the measurement of pH balance in saliva and urine as an objective means of monitoring this crucial aspect of physiology.

Author's note: Edgar Cayce, in some of his readings actually recommended consuming baking soda as a remedy for overacidity. So he beat me to my discovery. But I don't mind!

Chapter Ten

Alternative Cancer Therapies That Have Worked For Thousands

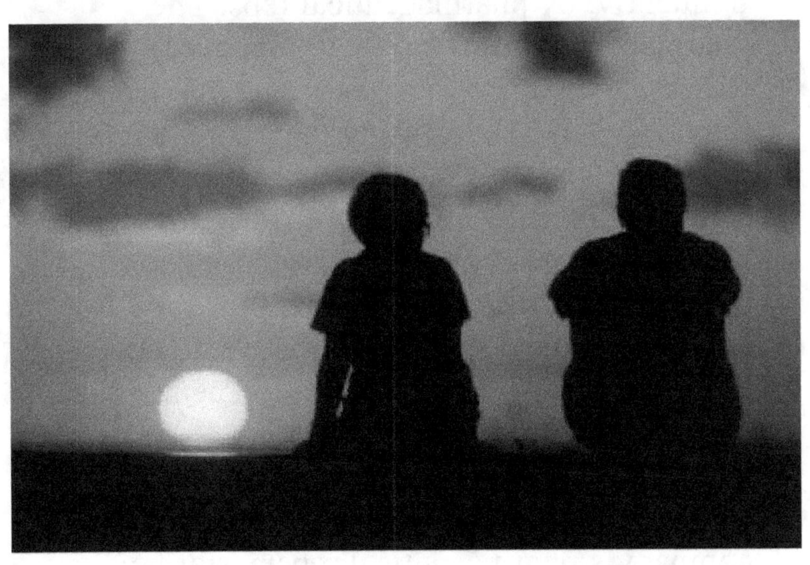

Seven Natural Cancer Remedies That Are Effective, Inexpensive, And Readily Available

Why You Should Read This

The typical practicing physician gets office visits from two categories of people. He gets visited by his patients, and typically he has a waiting room full of patients. He also gets visited, and frequently, by pharmaceutical reps. The pharmaceutical reps are there for several purposes. First, they are there as a reminder for the physician to keep using their company's drug products. But they are there also to brief the physician on their company's latest product developments. They will present the latest technical reports, and sales literature, and free samples, to the doctor. In this way each doctor keeps abreast of the latest developments in his field.

We all know how busy doctors are. The drug company's pharmaceutical reps perform a valuable service to the doctor, and the patients, by keeping the doctor fully informed and educated on the latest developments in the drug industry. The doctor does not have to go home at night and take part of his valuable and scarce private time to study about pharmaceutical advances; he is taught right in his office.

So when you come in to your doctor's office to report that you have cancer, the doctor is already up-to-date on the latest techniques advocated by the pharmaceutical companies for treating cancer. Is it any wonder then that this harried and overworked professional will prescribe a therapy to treat your cancer that follows the recommendations of the pharmaceutical companies? In addition, in medical school he was only taught cancer therapies that were approved by the American Medical Association that is heavily influenced and controlled by the pharmaceutical drug companies. Then, with his busy schedule, he just does not have the time or inclination to search out any natural and inexpensive cancer treatments that might serve you well.

This, of course, does not apply to all doctors. As awareness of the benefits of certain natural alternative cancer therapies become better known among the general populace, many brave doctors are venturing afield into holistic and natural medicines. But to do so places them at risk of censure and ridicule by their peers, as well as formal censure or loss of license to practice medicine.

The point I am making here is that your doctor, for one reason or another, may not tell you all that you need to know about the therapies which would best cure your cancer. So it may be up to you to seek out other sources of information, such as this book.

Those of you who may wish further information about the travails and misfortunes which may befall any doctor who "swims against the current" of conventional medical wisdom should search the Internet for the facts about Dr. Stanislaw Burzynski of Texas, who discovered a cure for certain types of cancer. He has been kept out of prison only because of the widespread support of many other brave physicians who have gone to bat for him. But his career and finances have been ruined because of persecution by the medical establishment. You may find an article about his situation on the Internet at .www.alkalizeforhealth.net/Lburzynski.htm.

There is a historical precedent for this type of situation. It took the medical establishment over fifty years to accept antibiotics! Yes, it is true. Penicillin, the first antibiotic, was discovered in the early 1890s. But the medical profession scoffed at the claims made about penicillin, and its use was ridiculed and scorned. It was not until World War II in the 1940s, when the medical profession was overwhelmed with the wounded and injured of war, that penicillin was tried on a mass scale and given a chance to prove its worth. The problem here is that you and I do not wish to wait fifty years for the medical establishment to approve natural effective remedies for cancer. We do not have the time.

Chapter Eleven
Oxygen Therapy

The cancer virus is anaerobic. This means that it can only live in the absence of oxygen. As a matter of fact, exposure to oxygen will kill this virus. The HIV virus is anaerobic. Exposure to oxygen will kill it. As a matter of fact, most disease causing viruses are anaerobic. They can only live where there is a low level of oxygen.

This fact becomes most interesting when it is noted that anaerobic viruses can only live in our body when the oxygen carrying capacity of our blood decreases to 60% of its optimum level. This has been known for some time. In 1931 Dr. Otto Warburg was awarded the Nobel Prize for Medicine for his discovery that he had found the cause of cancer to be a lack of oxygen at the cellular level. In 1953 the National Cancer

Institute endorsed Dr. Warburg's findings.
Additional observations:

Dr. Albert Wahl: "Disease is due to a deficiency
in the oxidation process of the body, leading to
an accumulation of toxins. These toxins are
ordinarily burned in normal oxidation."

Dr. Harry Goldblatt (<u>Journal of Experimental
Medicine</u>): "Lack of oxygen clearly plays a
major role in causing cells to become
cancerous."

Dr. Steven Levine: "Hypoxia, or the lack of
oxygen in the tissues, is the fundamental cause
of all degenerative diseases."

Dr. John Muntz: "Starved of oxygen the body
will become ill, and if this persists it will die. I
doubt that there is any argument about that."

There is clearly a correlation between the levels
of oxygen in our body and illness. It is important
to note that <u>fear, anxiety, worry, and depression</u>
all interfere with the breathing process, and will
reduce the oxygen intake. This can lead to
illness. But there is an even greater problem
facing our bodies and their needs for an adequate

supply of oxygen. It concerns the very air we breathe.

The Oxygen Story

Remember the movie Jurassic Park? In this movie, Scientists extracted DNA from the blood of mosquitoes, which were imbedded in fossilized amber in order to recreate prehistoric animals. Well, something similar has happened in real life. In the laboratory, real life scientists have extracted air, which was trapped as bubbles in fossilized amber. When the air was analyzed, it was found to contain 38% oxygen. This is very noteworthy because the air we breathe today has an average oxygen content of 21% or less.

The significance of this is immense. As man has evolved from his primitive prehistoric form, the oxygen levels of the air he breathes have dropped 50%. The implications of this on our health may be staggering. What if the human body was designed to live and prosper on air that contained 38% oxygen, a level that is 50% higher than the air we breathe today? What if the reduced levels of oxygen in the air we breathe today are causing our bodies to not receive an adequate level of oxygen for them to be well and healthy?

In fact, the air in various areas of the world is declining in oxygen content. In other words, this situation is getting worse. In some of the larger, more pollution plagued cities, the oxygen levels of air have declined as low as 15%. Man cannot live at levels at 7% oxygen or lower, even for a short period of time. It is safe to say that mankind may be facing a serious problem here.

Other Problems

We do not plan to go into great detail here about the other conditions in our lives, which result in our blood not carrying an adequate supply of oxygen to the muscles and cells of our bodies. In general, we have depleted our soils by the overuse of chemical fertilizers, resulting in our foodstocks not providing us with adequate nutrition. Example: Vegetables today have only 25% of the minerals and enzymes of vegetables grown 90 years ago. And many of the fruits and vegetables come to us contaminated with insecticides and pesticides. The consumption of processed salt, which has 82 of its 84 minerals and trace elements removed, and is coated with aluminum hydroxide which makes it insoluble in our bodies, harms our health. Most of the meat we consume today contains growth hormones and antibiotics, giving new meaning to the expression "you are what you eat." All of these factors lead to a lower level of overall health and energy, and a condition where our weakened bodies become overloaded with toxins. It is the job of our blood to extract these toxins from the cells of our bodies, and carry the toxins to the wall of the large intestine (colon). There the toxins are passed through the wall of the intestine, to be carried away with the waste products of our body.

But there is a problem here. The long-term consumption of too many processed foods has resulted in our large intestines becoming sluggish, which has led to a buildup on the intestinal walls of a hardened mucous-like coating. The average 50 year-old-American Male has a coating lining his colon, which weighs 5 pounds! It acts like a barrier between the wall of the large intestine (colon) and the waste products passing through the colon. As a result, the blood is not able to easily pass the toxins it is carrying through the wall of the colon. Unable to unload its toxins, the blood is forced to continue carrying the toxins. Under better conditions, the blood, after unloading its load of toxins, would pick up a load of oxygen to carry to the cells on its return trip. But now, still loaded with toxins, the blood is unable to carry oxygen back to the body's cells. Oxygen starvation results.

The Symptoms of Oxygen Deficiency

Doctors and scientists have identified the initial symptoms of oxygen deprivation, which actually constitutes the gradual oxygen starvation of the body's seven trillion cells. In addition to illness, these symptoms are:

• overall body weakness	• circulation problems
• muscle aches	• poor digestion
• depression	• lowered immunity to colds, flu, infection
• fatigue	• bronchial problems
• arthritis	• tumors and deposit buildups
• irrational behavior	• bacterial, viral and parasitic infestations

- irritability & dizziness
- memory loss
- hostility
- circulation problems
- acid stomach

People rarely suspect that the above conditions, or the constant vague feelings of helplessness, fatigue or despair is the result of the cells of their body desperately sending out signals that they need more oxygen.

The Use of Oxygen Therapies

By now I hope that I have convinced you of the need to get more oxygen to the cells of your body. You have probably surmised that if we could add oxygen directly to the blood in your body, most of the disturbing problems discussed above could be overcome. You are right. There are a number of ways to accomplish this. One approach is ozone therapy. Regular oxygen is O_2. Ozone is O_3, that is, each molecule has an extra atom of oxygen. When ozone is added to your body, the extra oxygen atom immediately leaves the ozone, and attached itself to a cell of your body. Your oxygen level is thereby increased. Chemically, the ozone (O3) has become oxygen (O2) plus oxygen (O). Ozone Therapy is widely practiced in other countries. In Germany, equipment and procedures have become refined to the point that doctors there can remove sluggish, toxin loaded blood from your body, ozonate the blood, remove the toxins, and reinsert the now oxygen enriched blood back into the patient's body. Other less complicated procedures involve using a relatively simple ozone machine to add ozone to the body through rectal insufflations, use of body wraps, or by simply drinking ozonated water. Wondrous cures for a wide litany of illnesses have been effected with ozone therapy. However, ozone therapy is not practiced in the United States.

Another procedure is the use of food grade hydrogen peroxide (H2O2). When hydrogen peroxide is added to the body, the H2O2 quickly becomes H2O (water) plus O (oxygen atom). The oxygen atom attaches itself to a cell of your body, and again, your oxygen level has just gone up. It is <u>very important</u> here to note that the type of hydrogen peroxide (3%), which is typically sold in drug stores and grocery stores, <u>cannot be used</u> for such a purpose. It contains contaminants and is dangerous for such use. Food Grade Hydrogen Peroxide (35%) is available through many health food stores. Food Grade Hydrogen Peroxide is the only type of hydrogen peroxide that can be used. Diluted Food Grade Hydrogen Peroxide can be given intravenously, or absorbed through the skin, or injested. One method which has successfully been used by many is to add 4 to 6 ounces of Food Grade 35% hydrogen peroxide to a tub of hot water and soak for 45 to 60 minutes. This is done daily. The hydrogen peroxide passes thru the skin into the blood stream where it is converted into oxygen. Miraculous recoveries from cancer, arthritis, Epstein Barr, chronic fatigue, lupus, multiple sclerosis, diabetes, allergies, and many other illnesses have been reported.

<u>Why Doesn't Your Doctor Tell You This?</u>

All oxygen therapies, including hydrogen peroxide therapy, are non-patentable processes. They are for the most part also inexpensive, and in many cases can be administered at home by the patient. Therefore there is no financial incentive for the pharmaceutical industry or the American Medical Association to promote these therapies. As a matter of fact, they will discipline severely any doctor caught using oxygen therapy.

This is not the case in certain other countries. In Germany, Russia, and Cuba, for example, physicians have successfully treated many serious and chronic conditions. Cancer, heart disease, AIDS, chronic fatigue, and many other illnesses have been successfully treated. In these countries a treatment consisting of a medical infusion of hydrogen peroxide costs approximately $10. No financial incentive here for the pharmaceutical industry, medical centers, and physicians who are accustomed to providing expensive drugs, and complex medical procedures. Thus, knowledge of this esoteric field is restricted to those intellectually courageous individuals who venture into the realms of alternative medicine.

What Can Be Done?

We have reviewed all of the oxygen therapy methods available, analyzed the cost and practicality of their application, and have reached a conclusion. Drinking water that contains a minute amount of food grade hydrogen peroxide is a good procedure. Many people have significantly increased the oxygen content of their blood, thereby improving their health or overcoming their illness, by this simple protocol. First of all, as we emphasize, use only 35% Food Grade Hydrogen Peroxide. Keep it in the refrigerator, or in a cool dark place (light will damage it). Use only distilled water, or reverse osmosis filtered water. This is because the iron content of regular water will react with the hydrogen peroxide to impart an unpleasant taste to the water. Carefully place 10 drops of the 35% hydrogen peroxide in an 8 oz. glass of distilled water, and immediately drink. Drink 5 glasses of this peroxide water daily. Best if taken on an empty stomach (it will taste better). That's it. Simple and cheap. And effective. Also, soaking daily in a tub of water to which 4 to 6 oz. of food grade hydrogen peroxide has been added, as already mentioned above, is a good therapy.

Mail Order Sources of Food Grade 35% Hydrogen Peroxide

First check with Google for an Internet source. Then check your local health food store. It may stock 35% food grade hydrogen peroxide. If not, you may obtain it from:

1. Sullivan Creek Distributing Co., 955 73rd Ave. NE. Carrington ND 58421, Toll Free Telephone: 888-406-4066, sells a 16 oz. bottle of food grade 35% hydrogen peroxide for $16.95.
2. Raw Health Inc., 11355 SW 14th St, Beaverton OR 97005, Telephone 866-729-4584, sells a 32 oz. bottle of food grade 35% hydrogen peroxide for $18.00.
3. Pure Health Systems, Telephone 970-731-9724 sells 35% food grade hydrogen peroxide. A 16 oz. bottle is $16.95 and a gallon bottle is $55.00.

Note: We are researchers, not physicians. Consult your physician. This researched information does not make any claims. It is not intended to replace sound medical advice.

<u>Additional Reading</u>

For additional reading, Crossroads, Toll Free Tel: 800-635-5823 sells books about oxygen therapy. I recommend *Oxygen Therapies* by Ed McCabe, and *Hydrogen Peroxide and Ozone* by Conrad LeBeau (only $3.95).

Bibliography

Oxygen by Dr. Kurt Donsbach, The Rockland Corporation, Tel: 800 421 7310

Bio/Tech News, newsletter, PO Box 30568, Parkrose Center, Portland OR 97294

Chapter Twelve

Essiac Tea: the Ojibwa Herbal Remedy from Canada

Essiac tea has a proven track record of curing thousands of cancer. Among its many reported properties, it attacks directly cancer tumors, detoxifies the body, removes heavy metals, and it builds up the immune system. It has also been found effective as a treatment for AIDS, lupus, chronic fatigue syndrome, diabetes, and many other illnesses. That such a simple remedy exists, is so widely unknown, and continues to be ignored by the mainstream medical establishment, is an amazing story.

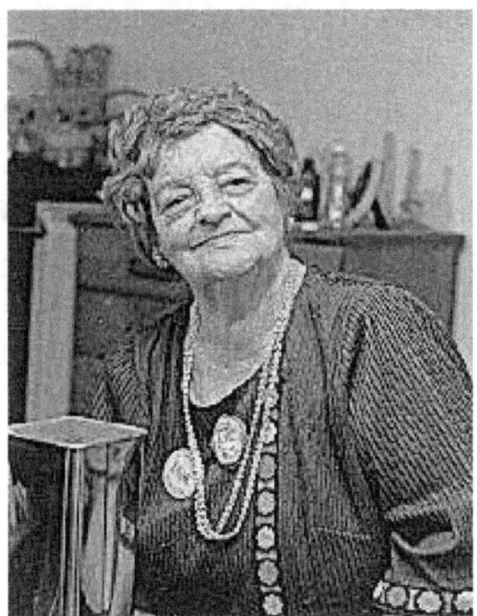

The Essiac Story:

Rene Caisse was a nurse in Canada. In 1923 she
observed that one of her doctor's patients, a
woman with terminal cancer, made a complete
recovery. Inquiring into the matter, Rene found
that the woman had used an herbal remedy given
to her by an Ojibway Indian herbalist. Rene
visited the Indian medicine man, and he gladly
and freely presented her with his tribe's formula.
He explained to her that the Ojibway used their
tonic both for spiritual balance and body healing.
The formula consisted of four common herbs.
They were blended and cooked in a fashion that
caused the concoction to have a greater curative
power than any of the four herbs themselves.
The four herbs were Sheep Sorrel, Burdock
Root, Slippery Elm Bark, and Rhubarb Root.

With her doctor's permission, Rene began to
administer the herbal remedy to other terminal
cancer patients who had been given up by the
medical profession as incurable. Most recovered.

Rene then began to collect the herbs herself,
prepare the remedy in her own kitchen, and to
treat hundreds of cancer cases. She set up a
clinic in Bracebridge, Ontario where she

administered the herbal remedy free to all who
sought her help. She found that Essiac, as she
named the herbal remedy, could not undo the
effects of severe damage to the life support
organs. In such cases, however, the pain of the
illness was alleviated and the life of the patients
was extended longer than predicted. In the other
cases, where the life support organs had not been
severely damaged, cure was complete, and the
patients lived another 35 or 40 years. Some are
still alive today.

Rene selflessly dedicated herself to helping these
patients. She continued to treat hundreds of
patients from her home. She did not charge for
her services. Donations were her only income.
They barely kept her above the poverty line.
Over the years word of her work began to
spread. The Canadian medical establishment did
not take kindly to this nurse administering this
remedy directly to anyone with cancer who
requested her help. Thus began many years of
harassment and persecution by the Canadian
Ministry of Health and Welfare. Word of this
struggle was carried throughout Canada by
newspapers.

The newspaper coverage of Rene's work began to make her famous. Word was also spread far and wide by the families of those healed by Essiac. Eventually, the Royal Cancer Commission became interested in her work. They undertook to study Essiac.

In 1937 the Royal Cancer Commission conducted hearings about Essiac. Eventually the Canadian Parliament, prodded by the newspaper coverage and the widespread support generated for Rene by former patients and grateful families, voted in 1938 on legislation to legalize the use of Essiac. Fifty-five thousand signatures were collected on a petition presented to the Parliament. The vote was close, but Essiac failed by three votes to be approved as an officially sanctioned cure for cancer.

Rene continued her work for 60 years. In the 1960s, Rene Caisse worked with the well-known Brusch Clinic in Massachusetts. Dr. Charles A. Brusch was the personal physician for President John F. Kennedy. After 10 years of research about Essiac, Dr. Brusch made the following statement: "Essiac is a cure for cancer, period. All studies done at laboratories in the United

States and Canada support this conclusion".
Rene Caisse died in 1978.

There are several excellent books about Essiac
Tea. I recommend "Essiac: A Native Herbal
Cancer Remedy" by Cynthia Olsen ($12.50) and
"Essiac Essentials: The Remarkable Herbal
Cancer Fighter" by Sheila Snow ($9.60). These
books may be ordered online at
.www.amazon.com or ordered from your local
bookstore.

What It Is

Rene Caisse's herbal formula contains four
commonly occurring herbs:

Sheep Sorrel (Rumex acetosella).

The leaves of young Sheep Sorrel plants were
popular as a cooking dressing and as an addition
to salads in France several hundred years ago.
Indians also use Sheep Sorrel leaves as a tasty
seasoning for meat dishes. They also baked it
into their bread. Thus it is both an herb and a
food.

Sheep Sorrel belongs to the buckwheat family. Common names for Sheep Sorrel are field sorrel, red top sorrel, sour grass and dog eared sorrel. It should not be confused with Garden Sorrel. (Rumex acetosa).

Sheep Sorrel grows wild throughout most of the world. It seeks open pastures, rocky areas, and the shoulders of country roads. It is considered to be a common weed throughout the U. S. The entire Sheep Sorrel plant may be harvested to be used in Essiac. Or, just the leaves and stems may be harvested, and this allows the plants to be "reharvested" later. The plant portion of the Sheep Sorrel may be harvested throughout the spring, summer, and fall. Harvest the leaves and stem before the flowers begin to form, since at this stage, all of the energy of the plant is in the leaves.

Burdock Root (Arctium lappa).

The roots, young stems, and seeds of the Burdock plant are edible. Young stalks are boiled to be eaten like asparagus. Raw stems and young leaves are eaten in salads. Parts of the Burdock plant are eaten in China, Hawaii, and among the Native American cultures on this continent. It is then, both an herb and a food.

The Burdock is a member of the thistle family. Remember the last time you cleaned cockleburs from your clothing after a sojourn in the woods or meadow? Chances are, you had run up against this very friendly and helpful plant, you just didn't know it! It is a common pasture weed throughout North America. It prefers damp soils. The first years the Burdock plant produces only green leafy growth. It is during the second year that it produces the long sturdy stems with annoying burrs.

The root of the Burdock plant is harvested. It is harvested from only the first year plants. The roots are about an inch wide, and up to three feet long. As with the Sheep Sorrel, the roots should only be harvested in the Fall when the plant energy is concentrated in the roots.

Slippery Elm (Ulcus fulva).

The inner bark of the Slippery Elm tree has a long history of use as a food supplement and herbal remedy. Pioneers knew of it as a survival food. The powdered bark has long been used, and is still being used today, as a food additive and food extender, rich in vitamin and mineral content. Thus it also is both an herb and a food. The Slippery Elm is a favorite shade and ornamental tree. It is found throughout Canada and the United States. Only the inner bark of the Slippery Elm is used to make Essiac.

Turkey Rhubarb (Rheum palmatum).

We have all eaten Rhubarb. Its red, bittersweet stems are to be found in supermarket produce shelves each spring. We also eat rhubarb pie, jams and pudding. The Turkey Rhubarb is a member of the rhubarb family with roots that contain a particularly strong and desirable potency.

The Turkey Rhubarb grows in China. The roots are harvested when the plants are at least six years old. This imported product has more potency than our native rhubarb. Rene Caisse began her Essiac work using the domestic rhubarb root, later discovering that the imported variety was more potent and less bitter. However most of the Turkey Rhubarb that is now imported into this country is irradiated, so that native rhubarb is now once again the rhubarb of choice.

<u>The Formula</u>

The original formula, as given by Rene Caisse, is listed below: Please note that she made large batches for many patients, and we are reprinting here her exact instructions for a two gallon batch, although you would probably not need such a large amount at one time.

Ingredients:
52 parts: Burdock Root (cut or dried) (parts by weight).
16 parts: Sheep Sorrel (powdered)
1 part: Turkey Rhubarb Root (powdered) or 2 parts native Rhubarb Root
4 parts: Slippery Elm Bark (powdered)

This is the basic four-herb formula that was presented to the Royal Cancer Commission in 1937 and was found by them to be a "cure for cancer". Later in her life, while working with Dr. Charles Brusch in Massachusetts, Rene added small potentizing amounts of four other herbs to her basic four-herb formula. They were added as follows: Kelp (2 parts), Red Clover (1 part), Blessed Thistle (1 part), Watercress (0.4 parts). I consider the addition of these four extra herbs optional.

Preparation: The above ingredients are boiled for ten minutes in two gallons of water. Then the mixture is allowed to cool and set for approximately 12 hours. Then it is reheated to boiling and strained and bottled.

Instructions for Use

1. Keep refrigerated.
2. Shake bottle well before using.
3. May be taken either cold from the bottle, or warmed (never microwave).
4. As a Preventative, daily take 4 tablespoons (2 ounces) at bedtime or on an empty stomach at least 2 hours after eating.
5. People with cancer and other people with health challenges may wish to twice daily take 4 tablespoons (2 ounces), once in the morning, 5

minutes before eating, and once in the evening, at least 2 hours after eating.

Note:

a. Stomach Cancer patients must dilute the herbal drink with an equal amount of sodium free distilled water.
b. Many people have reported that Rene's drink works well to detoxify the body, and have taken it as a detoxification program.
c. Precaution: Some doctors advise against taking the herbal formula while pregnant.

Recommendation: Rene reported that the twelve-hour brewing process is essential for Essiac to have its special powers. Essiac is now being offered to the public in pills, teabags, and homeopathic drops. We do not recommend them. They may work, but they are not what Rene used, nor have we seen evidence that they work.

What It Does

The components of Rene's herbal drink interact to have an amazing effect on the human body. The chemicals, minerals, and vitamins all act synergistically together to produce a variety of healing agents.

Sheep Sorrel:

Sorrel plants have been a folk remedy for cancer for centuries both in Europe and America. Sheep Sorrel has been observed by researchers to break down tumors, and to alleviate some chronic conditions and degenerative diseases.

It contains high amounts of vitamins A and B complex, C,D,E,K,P and vitamin U. It is also rich in minerals, including calcium, chlorine, iron, magnesium, silicon, sodium, sulphur, and has trace amounts of copper, iodine, manganese and zinc. The combination of these vitamins and minerals nourishes all of the glands of the body. Sheep Sorrel also contains carotenoids and chlorophyll, citric, malic, oxalic, tannic and tartaric acids.

The chlorophyll carries oxygen throughout the bloodstream. Cancer cells do not live in the presence of oxygen. It also:

• reduces the damage of radiation burns
• increases resistance to X-rays
• improves the vascular system, heart function, intestines, and lungs
• destroys parasites in the body
• aids in the removal of foreign deposits from the walls of the blood vessels
• purifies the liver, stimulates the growth of new tissue
• reduces inflammation of the pancreas, stimulates the growth of new tissue
• raises the oxygen level of the tissue cells

Sheep Sorrel is the primary healing herb in Essiac.

Burdock Root

For centuries Burdock has been used throughout the world to cure illness and disease. The root of the Burdock is a powerful blood purifier. It clears congestion in respiratory, lymphatic, urinary and circulatory systems. It promotes the flow of bile, and eliminates excess fluid in the body. It stimulates the elimination of toxic wastes, relieves liver malfunctions, and improves digestion. The Chinese use Burdock Root as an aphrodisiac, tonic, and rejuvenator. It assists in removing infection from the urinary tract, the liver, and the gall bladder. It expels toxins through the skin and urine. It destroys parasites. It is good against arthritis, rheumatism, and sciatica.

Burdock Root contains vitamins A, B complex, C, E, and P. It contains high amounts of chromium, cobalt, iron, magnesium, phosphorus, potassium, silicon, and zinc. It also contains smaller amounts of calcium, copper, manganese, selenium, and sulphur.

Much of the Burdock Root's curative power is attributed to its principal ingredient of Unulin, which helps to strengthen vital organs, especially the liver, pancreas, and spleen.

Slippery Elm Inner Bark

Slippery Elm Bark is widely known throughout the world as an herbal remedy. As a tonic it is known for its ability to sooth and strengthen the organs, tissues, and mucous membranes, especially the lungs and stomach. It promotes fast healing of cuts, burns, ulcers and wounds. It revitalizes the entire body.

It contains, as its primary ingredient, a mucilage, as well as quantities of gallic acid, phenols, starches, sugars, the vitamins A, B complex, C, K, and P. It contains large amounts of calcium, magnesium, and sodium, as well as lesser amounts of chromium and selenium, and trace amounts of iron, phosphorous, silicon and zinc.

Slippery Elm Bark is known among herbalists for its ability to cleanse, heal, and strengthen the body.

Rhubarb Root

Rhubarb, also a well-known herb, has been used worldwide since 220 BC as a medicine.

The Rhubarb root exerts a gentle laxative action by stimulating the secretion of bile into the intestines. It also stimulates the gall duct to expel toxic waste matter, thus purging the body of waste bile and food. As a result, the liver is cleansed, and chronic liver problems are relieved.

Rhubarb root contains vitamin A, many of the B complex, C, and P. Its high mineral content includes calcium, chlorine, copper, iodine, iron, magnesium, manganese, phosphorous, potassium, silicon, sodium, sulphur, and zinc.

Reported Benefits of Essiac:

1. Prevents the buildup of excess fatty deposits in artery walls, heart, kidney and liver.

2. Regulates cholesterol levels by transforming sugar and fat into energy.
3. Destroys parasites in the digestive system and throughout the body.
4. Counteracts the detrimental effects of aluminum, lead and mercury poisoning.
5. Strengthens and tightens muscles, organs and tissues.
6. Makes bones, joints, ligaments, lungs, and membranes strong and flexible, less vulnerable to stress or stress injuries.
7. Nourishes and stimulates the brain and nervous system.
8. Promotes the absorption of fluids in the tissues.
9. Removes toxic accumulations in the fat, lymph, bone marrow, bladder, and alimentary canals.
10. Neutralizes acids, absorbs toxins in the bowel, and eliminates both.
11. Clears the respiratory channels by dissolving and expelling mucus.
12. Relieves the liver of its burden of detoxification by converting fatty toxins into water-soluble substances that can then be easily eliminated through the kidneys.
13. Assists the liver to produce lecithin, which forms part of the myelin sheath, a white fatty

material that encloses nerve fibers.
14. Reduces, perhaps eliminates, heavy metal deposits in tissues (especially those surrounding the joints) to reduce inflammation and stiffness.
15. Improves the functions of the pancreas and spleen by increasing the effectiveness of insulin.
16. Purifies the blood.
17. Increases red cell production, and keeps them from rupturing.
18. Increases the body's ability to utilize oxygen by raising the oxygen level in the tissue cells.
19. Maintains the balance between potassium and sodium within the body so that the fluid inside and outside each cell is regulated: in this way, cells are nourished with nutrients and are also cleansed.
20. Converts calcium and potassium oxalates into a harmless form by making them solvent in the urine. It also regulates the amount of oxalic acid delivered to the kidneys, thus reducing the risk of stone formation in the gall bladder, kidneys, or urinary tract.
21. Protects against toxins entering the brain.
22. Protects the body against radiation and X-rays.
23. Relieves pain, increases appetite, and provides more energy along with giving a sense of well-being.

24. Speeds up wound healing by regenerating the damaged area.
25. Increases the production of antibodies like lymphocytes and T-cells in the thymus gland, which is the defender of our immune system.
26. Inhibits and possibly destroys benign growths and tumors.
27. Protects the cells against free radicals.

An Endorsement by Dr. Julian Whitaker, M.D.

Dr. Julian Whitaker publishes a very informative and enlightening monthly newsletter named *Health and Healing*. It has 430,000 subscribers. In his November 1995 issue, he had an article entitled "What I Would Do If I Had Cancer". He states that if he had cancer he personally would follow a regime that included <u>Essiac Tea</u>.

Dr. Whitaker has over twenty years' experience. He has written five major health books: *Reversing Heart Disease, Reversing Diabetes, Reversing Health Risks, A Guide to Natural Healing* and *Is Heart Surgery Necessary?* Dr. Whitaker directs the Whitaker Wellness Institute in Newport Beach, California, which has treated thousands of patients. Should you desire information about subscribing to his newsletter, call (800) 705-5559.

I highly recommend this newsletter to anyone who has a serious illness and wishes to become more knowledgeable about the complete range of healing modalities available. He also proscribes a 7-step, 30-day wellness program "that will turn your life around."

Quotes from Rene Caisse:

"Though I worked each day from 9am to 9pm, my work was so absorbing there was no sense of fatigue. My waiting room was a place of happiness where people exchanged their experiences and shared their hope. After a few treatments, patients seemed to throw off their depression, fear and distress. Their outlook became optimistic and as their pain decreased, they became happy and talkative."

"I could see the changes in some of the patients. A number of them, presented to me by their doctors after everything known to medical science had been tried and failed, were literally carried into my clinic for their first treatment. To later see these same people walk in on their own, after only five or six treatments, more than repaid me for all my endeavours. I have helped thousands of such people. I offered the treatment at no charge."

"Most importantly, and this was verified in animal tests conducted at the Brusch Medical Centre and other laboratories, it was discovered that one of the most dramatic effects of taking this remedy was its affinity for drawing all of the cancer cells which had spread, back to the original site at which point the tumour would first harden, then later soften until it vanished altogether. In other cases, the tumour would decrease in size to where it could be surgically removed with minimal complications."

Source List of Suppliers

I recommend Natural Heritage Enterprises, PO Box 278, Crestone CO 81131, Toll Free Telephone: 888-568-3036. They sell Essiac Tea in bottles and also in a less expensive package of dried herbs for those who wish to brew their own tea. I like their bonus buy: purchase 12 and get 6 additional for free (18 bottles of tea or 18 packages of herbs for the price of 12).

Bottles: Bottles of the herbal remedy can be purchased by mail order for $14.50 per 16 oz. bottle (a 4 day supply).

Dried Herbal Mix: Should you wish to prepare your own Essiac herbal drink, you may mail order packets of the dried herb combination. Each packet will allow you to prepare approximately one half gallon of the drink (a two week supply). The cost is $12.00 per packet.

Essiac Testimonials

CHARLES A BRUSCH, M.D.
15 GROZIER ROAD

CAMBRIDGE, MA 02138

TO WHOM IT MAY CONCERN:

Many years have gone by since I first experienced the use of ESSIAC with my patients who were suffering from many varied forms of cancer.

I personally monitored the use of this old therapy along with Rene Caisse R.N., whose many successes were widely reported. Rene worked with me at my medical clinic in Cambridge, Massachusetts where, under the supervision of 18 of my medical doctors on staff, she proceeded with a series of treatments on terminal cancer patients and laboratory mice. Together we refined and perfected her formula.

On mice it has been shown to cause a decided recession of the mass and a definite change in cell formation. Clinically, on patients suffering from

pathologically proven cancer, it
reduces pain and causes a
recession in growth. Patients
gained weight and showed a great
improvement in their general
health. Their elimination
improved considerably and their
appetite became whetted.

Remarkably beneficial results
were obtained even on those
cases at the "end of the road",
where it proved to prolong life
and the "quality" of that life.
In some cases, if the tumour
didn't disappear, it could be
surgically removed after ESSIAC
with less risk of metastases
resulting in new outbreaks.

Hemorrhage has been rapidly
brought under control in many
difficult cases, open lesions of
lip and breast respond to
treatment, and patients with
cancer of the stomach have
returned to normal activity
among many other remembered
cases. Also, intestinal burns
from radiation were healed and

damage replaced, and it was
found to greatly improve
whatever the condition.

All the patient cases were
diagnosed by reputable
physicians and surgeons. I do
know that I have witnessed in my
clinic, and know of many other
cases, where ESSIAC was the
therapy used - a treatment which
brings about restoration through
destroying the tumour tissue and
improving the mental outlook
which re-establishes
physiological function.

I endorse this therapy even
today for I have in fact cured
my own cancer, the original site
of which was the lower bowel,
through ESSIAC alone. My last
complete examination, when I was
examined throughout the
intestinal tract while
hospitalized (August, 1989) for
a hernia problem, revealed no
sign of malignancy. Medical
documents validate this. I have
taken ESSIAC every day since my

diagnosis (1984) and my recent examination has given me a clear bill of health.

I remained a partner with Rene Caisse until her death in 1978 and was the only person who had her complete trust and to whom she confided her knowledge and "know-how" of what she named "ESSIAC."

Others have imitated, but a minor success rate should never be accepted when the true therapy is available.

Executed as a legal document.

Signed: Charles A. Brusch, M.D., April 11, 1990

Editor's note: Dr. Brusch was JFK's personal physician

Other Endorsements:

My research company has investigated cancer
and the cancer industry for over 12 years.
During this time, we have had the opportunity to
examine many alternative treatments for cancer
in great detail. I do not hesitate to recommend
Essiac products to the public as part of the
metabolic therapy support program for the
prevention of, and treatment for all types of
cancer. Essiac is covered in my best-selling
book, Cancer: Why We're Still Dying to Know
the Truth, available through Credence
Publications.

Phillip Day

Health Reporter

Credence Research, UK

Chapter Thirteen

Kombucha the Amazing Mushroom Tea

Years ago the Russian government sent a team of investigators to check out why the residents of an area in Manchuria were cancer free. The people of this area also regularly lived to be over 100 years of age. After a two-year study, the investigators attributed the longevity and good health of these people to a yeast enzyme tea called Kombucha. It had been part of their diet for hundreds of years. Now the use of Kombucha has been spreading like wildfire in the United States.

In an April, 1995 issue of <u>US Today</u> newspaper, an article about Kombucha tea stated that five to six million Americans were drinking Kombucha tea daily. I am sure that this number of Kombucha drinkers has grown since then. It is inexpensive, I find it fun to make, and most people enjoy the taste. I keep several one gallon "sun tea" jars of Kombucha brewing at all times. I keep the jars prominently sitting on my kitchen counter, where they become a conversation piece for my visitors.

During an August, 1995 TV program of <u>Entertainment Tonight</u> which covered Kombucha, it was mentioned that the Hollywood stars Cher, Susan Sarandon, Martin Landau, Meg Ryan and Linda Evans were all Kombucha drinkers. In addition, Anjelica Huston, Lily Tomlin, Morgan Fairchild, and Rita Coolidge are said to be Kombucha fans. It is

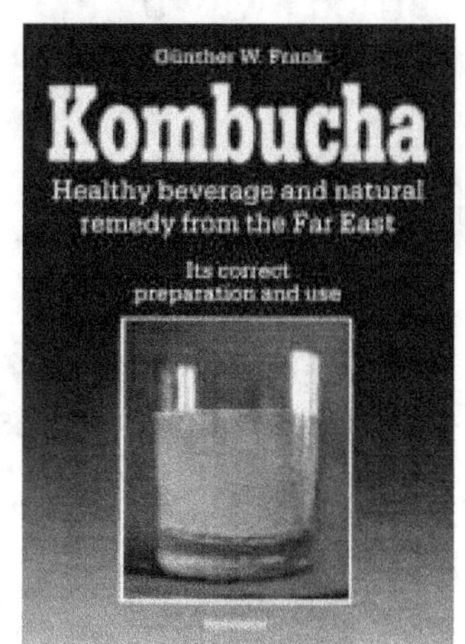

reported that Kombucha cleanses the blood, stops cancer, increases energy levels, reverses hardening of the arteries, reduces high blood pressure, boosts T-cell counts, removes wrinkles, thickens the hair, and relieves headaches. Studies in California report that HIV patients drinking Kombucha do not progress into

AIDS. Other testimonials state that it reverses
graying hair, stops PMS, reverses the symptoms
of multiple sclerosis, and shrinks prostates.

Kombucha is known to provide the liver with
glucuronic acid, a substance that the liver uses to
detoxify our bodies. In this manner, Kombucha
helps the liver to perform its critical function of
"binding up" toxic substances so they can be
carried away by the blood and dispelled from
our bodies.

Amazom.com on the Internet sells a number of
books about Kombucha. There is also the book
**"Kombucha: Healthy Beverage and Natural
Remedy from the Far East"** by Guenther Frank
which can be purchased from Pronatura, Inc. at
847-545-1003.

Kombucha has been around for centuries
without causing any known widespread ill
effects. Although newly discovered in the
United States, there has been plentiful research
done in Europe and Asia confirming its healthful
benefits. Kombucha is fun to make, tastes great,
is cheap, and if you take it daily, you too may
live to become 100 years old.

Sources of a Kombucha Starter Kit

1. Mt. Nebo Herbs & Oils, 300 Highland Ave., Athens OH 45701, Tel: 740-592-3795 sells a Kombucha starter kit, including Kombucha mushroom and full instructions for $15.50 plus $6.95 for Shipping.

2. 2. Laurel Farms, PO Box 2896, Sarasota FL 34230, Tel: 941-351-2233 sells a Kombucha starter kit, including Kombucha mushroom and full instructions, for $39.00 including Shipping and Handling.

3. Nancy Adams, Ph.D., Tel: 541-888-5111, sells a Kombucha starter kit for $15.00 including Shipping.

Note: These starter kits are all that you will need to produce a lifetime supply of Kombucha tea.

Chapter Fourteen

Pycnogenol and Grape Seed Extract

An excess of free radicals in a person's body causes major damage, including cancer. Free radicals can attack, damage, and ultimately destroy any material including the sensitive cells and tissues in the body. The best free radical killer is Pycnogenol (pronounced pig-nodge-a-nol). Pycnogenol is a patented antioxidant from France that is made from a pine tree bark extract.

Let's talk more about free radicals. The normal oxygen atom in your body has four pairs of electrons. However the effects of radiation, sunlight, air pollution, harmful chemicals, food additives, tobacco smoke, infections and

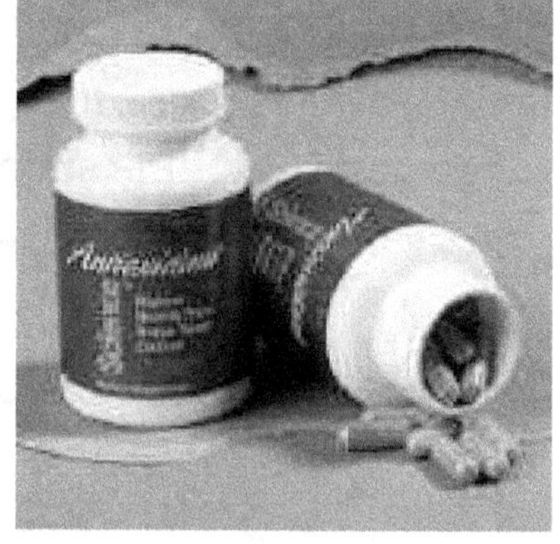

stress can rob one of the electrons from the oxygen atom. This atom is now a free radical. It tries to replace its lost electron by raiding other molecules. It will rob an electron from a molecule in a cell wall. This robbed molecule proceeds to replace its lost electron by robbing another molecule, and a chain reaction is created. This leads to disintegration of the cell, and opens the door to cancer and many other ills. It also alters the DNA which damages the way in which the cells in your body replicate. This leads to aging. Some studies suggest that these free radicals are a major cause of aging.

How does Pycnogenol help? It is a very powerful antioxidant. An antioxidant has extra electrons that it can "give up" to the free radicals, thereby rendering them harmless.

I recommend Pycnogenol because of its power. It has the ability, in a matter of a few months, to destroy all of the excess free radicals that you have built up over a lifetime. It is inexpensive. It is easy to locate. It comes in tablet form. Every health food store stocks it. Dr. Lamar Rosquist recommends that you take one mg. of Pycnogenol daily per pound of body weight during the initial period when you are ridding yourself of all accumulated free radicals. This means that a 200 pound man would take 200 mg. of Pycnogenol daily for the first two or three months. Later you may wish to slack off to a lower maintenance-level dosage.

Pycnogenol is reported to assist in the recovery of cancer, Alzheimers, arthritis, Parkinsons, rheumatism, asthma, diabetes, stress, varicose veins, phlebitis, PMS, AIDS, senility, M.S., chronic fatigue, stroke, circulatory and cardiovascular problems. It adds energy. It has also been reported to greatly assist in limiting wrinkling and aging of the skin.

When I took Pycnogenol, I found my energy levels dramatically boosted.

Grape Seed Extract is reportedly as good as Pycnogenol as a free radical killer. To locate a source of Pycnogenol or Grape Seed Extract, I suggest that you visit one or more health food stores. They may be able to offer some helpful advice, and they may have literature available with additional information about this antioxidant. I have even found Pycnogenol and Grape Seed Extract stocked in K Mart and my local drug store.

Sources of Pycnogenol and Grape Seed Extract

Nature's Rx, 119 Spinnaker Circle, Madison AL 35758, Toll Free Tel: 800-303-5781 sells Grape Seed Extract. A bottle of 90 caplets (90mg per cap) costs $12.00.

Nutri Team, Ripton VT 05766, Toll Free Tel: 800-785-9791 sells Grape Seed Extract. A bottle of 120 caplets (100 mg per cap) costs $11.95.

Primary Source, Inc., PO Box 812, Fairfield CT 06430, Toll Free Tel: 888-666-1188 sells a product named OPC that contains both Pycnogenol and grape seed extract. A bottle of 60 caplets (100 mg per cap) costs $44.95.

Chapter Fifteen
Colon Health and Cancer

Almost everyone remembers that John Wayne died of cancer. When an autopsy was performed on him, it was found that his colon (large intestine) was six inches in diameter and weighed 60 pounds empty. The hole in the center of the colon through which his food passed was one inch in diameter. The large intestine of the average person is about 5 feet long, and is 2.5 inches in diameter. John Wayne's enlarged colon was so packed with an accumulation of undigested and solidified food that there was no way in which he could have lived. I say that John Wayne died of an unhealthy colon, because cancer is only one of the results of an unhealthy and blocked colon. One of the functions of the blood in your body is to carry oxygen and nutrients to each cell in your body. The blood, after delivering this oxygen and nutrition to each cell, then picks up the waste product of the cell and carries it to the wall of the colon. There the waste products are passed through the wall of the colon, to be carried out of the body with the next bowel movement. However, if the interior walls of the colon have become coated with solidified food and waste, this coating on the wall of the colon will block the passage of the blood's load of waste products. Thus, this function of passing the blood's load of cell waste cannot be performed. The blood, not able to unload its load of waste products, will begin to carry it around the body. Loaded down with this load of toxic waste products, the blood is not able to pick up a full load of oxygen and nutrients to resupply the body's cells. Starved of the necessary oxygen and nutrients, the body's cells begin to deteriorate.

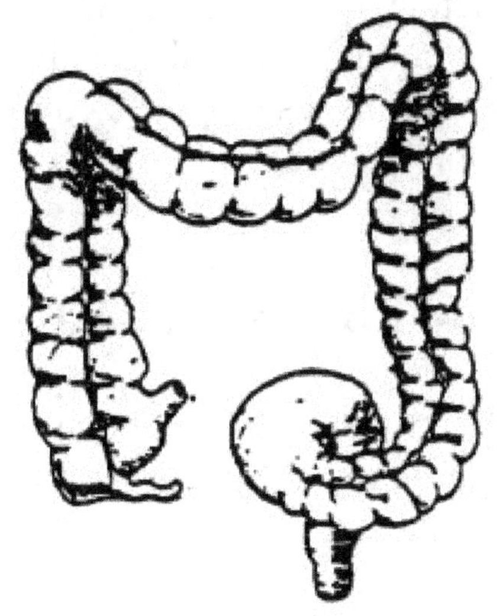

This leads to a host of unhealthy conditions, including eventually cancer. Remember, in Chapter 1 we discussed that cancer can only exist in an environment where there is a lack of oxygen. So it is that the state of health of your large intestine (colon) has a lot to do with whether or not you get cancer.

It is a medical fact that the average American male has a coating of solidified food lining the inside walls of his colon which weighs five pounds! How does this happen? A lifetime of eating too many fatty foods, a diet not containing enough fiber, and too many processed foods in our diet are the culprits. The eventual result of our years of improper eating is that deposits begin to accumulate on the walls of the colon, eventually leading to serious health situations, as emphasized by the example of John Wayne.

Symptoms of an Unhealthy Colon

As we get older, we begin to experience the symptoms of aging. But many times, these are not the symptoms of the normal aging process, they are symptoms of a plugged up colon. We just mistake them as signs of the normal aging process. Symptoms of an unhealthy colon are:

Fatigue	Depression	Anxiety or worry
Gas or Flatulence	Protruding Abdomen	Insomnia
Not feeling good	Lack of interest	Abdominal discomfort
Headaches	Aches and pains	Menstrual problems
Irritability	Loss of memory	Skin problems
Nervousness	Overweight	Bad breath
Nausea	Craving for food	Feel cold (hands and feet)
Swelling of the legs	Disinterest in sex	

What Can Be Done?

Obviously, changing your diet to minimize fats and processed foods, and adding fiber, will be required in order to correct the conditions of an unhealthy colon. But if you have cancer, you cannot afford to wait for the months or years it may take to correct the problem. You need to fix your colon now. The answer is Colonics.

What is a Colonic?

A Colonic is much like an enema, except that it is much more thorough and effective. In a 45-minute session, approximately 15 gallons of water is used to gently flush the colon. Through appropriate use of massage, pressure points, etc., the colon therapist is able to work loose and eliminate far more toxic waste than any other short-term technique.

What will Colonics do for the colon ?

Specifically, a Colonic is used to accomplish the
following:

1.It cleanses the Colon: Toxic material is
broken down so it can no longer harm your
body or inhibit assimilation and elimination.
Even debris built up over a long period is
gently, but surely removed in the process of a
series of treatments. Once impacted material
is removed, your colon can begin again to co-
operate as it was intended to. In this very real
sense a colonic is a rejuvenation treatment.

2. It Exercises the Colon Muscles: The build up
of toxic debris weakens the colon and impairs
it's functioning. The gentle filling and emptying
of the colon improves peristaltic (muscular
contraction) activity by which the colon
naturally moves material.

3. It Reshapes the Colon: When problem
conditions exist in the colon, they tend to alter
its shape which in turn causes more problems.
The gentle action of the water, coupled with the
massage techniques of the colon therapist helps
to eliminate bulging pockets of waste and

narrowed, spastic constrictions. This enables the colon to resume its natural state.

4. It Stimulates Reflex Points: Every system and organ of the body is connected to the colon by reflex points. A colonic stimulates these points, thereby affecting the corresponding body parts in a beneficial way.

When the lower intestinal tract is cleansed, the whole system is detoxified. Proponents of colon irrigation claim that it actually heals their bodies. Toxicity is a major cause of illness, disease and feelings of general malaise. While colon therapy does not heal any specific disease, it greatly enhances the body's ability to function at optimum levels, so the body is more able to heal itself.

When a system has experienced abusive treatment it has had to endure over a lifetime, toxic waste builds up in the colon and the body cannot properly assimilate the vitamins and minerals we need. The walls of the colon tend to develop a buildup of material and this results in sluggish bowel movements, constipation and other problems. Instead of being expelled correctly, the poisons re-enter the blood stream and circulate through the body. If you are experiencing flatulence, stomach bloat, lower backache, bad breath, stiff joints, mood swings, skin problems, abdominal discomfort, restless sleep, excessive mucous, nausea, constipation, diarrhea, fatigue depression or cloudy urine, you may need to have your colon cleansed. These are signs of an impacted colon.

Many people are under the false impression that an enema is as cleansing as a colonic. An enema only uses 1 to 2 quarts of water while colonic irrigation uses 12 to 15 gallons of water. During the colonic the water travels the whole 5-foot length of the colon, cleaning it from the sigmoid to the ascending colon. The whole colonic treatment is not necessarily limited to the colonic irrigation. Also included usually is abdominal massage and reflexology that is used to stimulate pressure points of the feet that also help with the elimination process. The entire procedure should take 35 to 40 minutes.

The effect of a colonic is not just on the colon. Once your body is detoxified through the colonic irrigation, the other organs of the body work better. It facilitates the cleansing of the blood, liver and the lymphatic system and makes it easier for organs to release their waste products for elimination. Many people claim they suffer from headaches much less after having a colonic treatment. Other benefits that are reported are improvement in appearance, mental attitude, skin tone, and stress is relieved. Constipation and abdominal pain are often eliminated and the old feeling of exhaustion is replaced with a feeling of energy. And if you have cancer, the glands and organs of your body will function better, causing your immune system to work better, and be able to better combat the cancer in your body.

Where Can I Get a Colonic?

Good places to locate a colon therapist who will administer a colonic are your local health food store bulletin board and the telephone book yellow pages. You may also wish to ask about among the health-conscious. One of them will be able to recommend a good colonics specialist to you.

Chapter Sixteen

Cancer and the Parasite Connection

Dr Hulda Clark is a medical researcher from Canada. She is convinced that many diseases, especially cancer, result from the invasion of parasites in the colon.

From this simply stated but well researched idea, she has written a series of books and produced a range of products and recommendations which have resulted in a huge following in the United States of America and in many other countries.

Her first best selling book " The Cure for all Cancers" has been followed by "The Cure for all Diseases", and she has developed her ideas and her following by the good results her patients are experiencing. Dr Clark believes that if the body can be rid of colon parasites it can restore itself to full health. Dr Clark recommends a

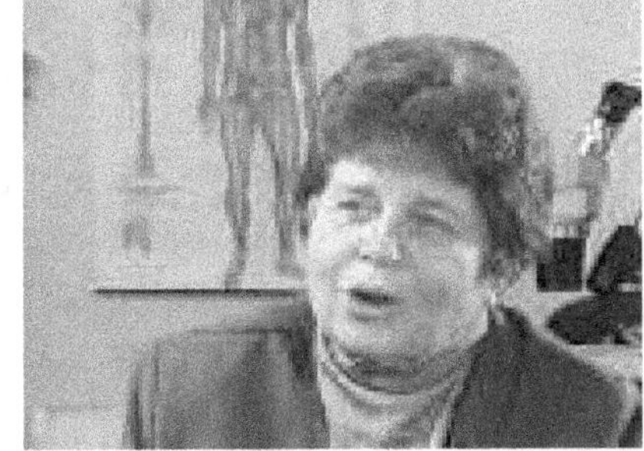

combination of herbal parasite cleanses, the use of her inexpensive electronic "zapper", and kidney and liver flushes as the best possible ways to rid the body of colon parasites.

How is it that a parasite can cause cancer?

Unknown to most of us, most people have one or more types of parasites in their bodies. They got them from running barefoot as children, from eating undercooked meat, from eating improperly washed fruits and vegetables, and from handling pets. One of these parasites is an intestinal fluke. Its scientific name is *Fasciolopsis buskli*. It is quite small. Normally this fluke lives in our intestinal tract, where it does little harm. But sometimes, over years without detection or treatment, these flukes multiply to the point where they begin to travel outside the colon to other parts of the body. Sometimes they invade other organs or parts of the body. There they do a great deal of harm. There they can cause cancer.

For example, let us assume a situation where these intestinal flukes have invaded and established themselves in a liver. There they multiply until there may be thousands of flukes. These flukes are all busy devouring your body fluids and nutrients, and in turn spewing out their waste products. These waste products

contaminate your liver. There is a growth factor in your
liver that is called ortho-phospo-tyrosine. For
brevity I shall refer to it as "ortho". This ortho
has a normal function of causing cells to divide.
But the fluke's waste products cause the ortho to
sometimes go haywire, and the ortho causes
cells to divide where they shouldn't. This leads
to improperly growing cells, which often leads
to cancer.

Why Cancer Locates Where It Does

Why does one person develop cancer in the
lungs, and another person develop cancer in the
kidneys? It is because this particular area of the
body is weakened. Generally, parasites thrive
better in a weakened organism. So the flukes
will be attracted to this weakened area of the
body. Eventually a cancerous condition will
develop.

Why is this particular part of the body
weakened? Because it probably has a number of
the following problems:

a. has low immune   d. receives improper

power

b. accumulated a heavy dosage of heavy metals

c. accumulated a large dosage of toxins

nutrition

e. does not receive enough oxygen

f. has too many free radicals.

Let's Get Rid Of The Parasites!

Dr. Hulda Clark recommends the following protocols to get rid of the parasites in your body:

1. A Herbal Parasite Cleanse. Dr. Clark recommends a combination of Black Walnut Hull extract, Wormwood and Cloves. My favorite source for these parasite-removing products is the company founded by Hanna Kroeger, a famous herbalist. It is Kroeger Herbal Products, 805 Walnut St., Boulder CO 80302, Toll Free Tel: 800-516-0690. Tell them what you wish to do, and they will advise which products to buy and how to take them. They are very honest people.
2. The "Zapper". Dr Clark discovered that a minute electrical charge, at a certain frequency, will kill all of the parasites

without harming the body. She has developed an inexpensive device named the "Zapper" which will do this. She provides complete construction details and schematics in her book *The Cure For All Cancers*. All parts can be bought at Radio Shack. However if you are as electronically illiterate as I am, I suggest that you buy a Zapper from one of the many small companies that supply them to the public. You may wish to call:

    a. Essence Instruments, 119 Pearl St., Kingston NY 12401, Toll Free Tel: 877-317-3341. Cost is $65.00

    b. Transformation Technologies, PO Box 2698, North Hills CA 91393, Toll Free Tel: 877-287-0712. Cost is $80.00

    c. Sota Instruments, PO Box 2698, Revelstoke BC, Canada, North America Toll Free Tel: 800-224-0242. Cost is $83.00.

3. Liver and Kidney Flushes. She also gives detailed instructions in her book on how to give yourself a liver and kidney flush. I have done these flushes on a number of occasions. They cost almost nothing, take only a day, and give only the mildest

discomfort. In short, they are a breeze. You will feel in much better health after taking them.

The Book

If this parasite information is of interest to you, you definitely should take the plunge and buy the book **The Cure For All Cancers** by Dr. Hulda Clark, MD. The normal retail price is $21.95. If your local health food store does not stock the book, you can order it at .ww.amazon.com, or you may contact Spirit of Healing, 144 N. Cherry St, #7, Kernersville NC 27284, Toll Free Tel: 877-275-3196.

Other Doctor's Comments

"It is Dr. Clark's merit to have discovered the fact that parasitic burdens play a central role in cancer." -- Dr. Alan Baklayan, Orthomolecular Medicine, Munich, Germany

"We have a tremendous parasite problem right here in the United States-it's just not being identified."
-Peter Weina, Ph.D., Chief of Pathobiology, Walter Reed Army Institute of Research, 1991

"I strongly believe that every patient with disorders of immune function, including multiple allergies (especially food allergy), and patients with unexplained fatigue or with chronic bowel symptoms should be evaluated for the presence of intestinal parasites."
-Leo Galland, M.D. Townsend Letter for Doctors, 1988

"Make no mistake about it, worms are the most toxic agents in the human body. They are one of the primary underlying causes of disease and are the most basic cause of a compromised immune system."
-Hazel Parcells, D.C., N.D., Ph.D., 1974

Testimonials

Cancer Testimonial #1

On October 8, 1998, at age 55, I was diagnosed with cutaneous T Cell Lymphoma. I was given a few months to live. A bone marrow was done and a catscan was taken four days later, coincident with the commencement of chemotherapy. A week later, the results of the bone marrow and catscan indicated a more promising prognosis -- I could live another five years. Five months of chemotherapy ensued.

At the end of the chemotherapy (February), my oncologist and I were pleased with the results. Chemo was done! He would see me again in three months.

Unfortunately in mid April, the lymphoma returned. The largest tumor was removed but two more tumors grew. The doctors felt that neither chemo nor surgery would work so they decided to try radiation. In Canada, we have a waiting period to try radiation so it was booked for July.

I was terrified of having radiation and decided to pursue Hulda Clark's book, the Cure for All Cancers, which I had bought during my chemotherapy sessions. Commencing with the daily kidney cleanse tea, and then adding the parasite cleanse, I followed the regimen in her book. Three weeks later, the tumors were gone!

On July 7, I met with the radiologist as it was a consultation only. He examined me and said, you don't need radiation, you look great. He also confirmed that radiation, as it is a 'spot' treatment, would not get all the cancer, only certain tumors. He was very interested in the cleanses I was taking and researched the ingredients while I was at the hospital. His conclusion was they were doing me no harm, in fact 'wormwood' is known in medical circles to kill tumors and advised he would render a report to my oncologist. The radiologist recommended a kidney test to ensure the cleanse was not toxic to my kidneys; however, he felt the dose was too minimal to be toxic.

August 9, I saw my oncologist and after several blood and kidney tests, was told I did not need to see him again, I could expect to live a 'normal life expectancy', I was fine! We have jointly agreed to checkups every 3 months as a preventative measure. Interestingly, I showed him a bottle of the parasite cleanse and he said I was the second of his patients to show him the cleanse, the other patient had leukemia, and was doing as well as I.

October 2, I returned from two weeks, touring, hiking and exploring the Canadian Rockies. I feel great, thanks to Hulda Clark.

I realize that testimonials can be 'a dime a dozen' but having been diagnosed with what we all dread, Cancer, I decided early in my diagnosis that I had to take control of my healing and exhaust all opportunities -- dying was never on my agenda. What did I have to lose, nothing and I had my life to gain. My two daughters thought I was crazy to do the cleanse but support it wholeheartedly now. There are many of us taking the cleanse and doing well, some who have refused all 'conventional medical' treatment (chemotherapy and radiation).

I think I owe my life to Hulda Clark's parasite cleanse.

Sincerely,
CT

Cancer Testimonial #2

We just received the great news that JL is cured of cancer! You might remember her -- she is 30 years of age and was suffering from Stage 3 brain cancer. Chemo was failing her since there was new growth after the chemo treatments. She has written you and was closely following the parasite cleanse and using the zapper. She went to a local clinic for a body scan and she was told that he couldn't pick up any evidence that she had cancer. Therefore, she had her M.D. schedule a special test in Phoenix in hopes that the medical community would agree with the alternative therapist. Sure enough, results just came back that the growth of her tumor was not only retarded but she showed no evidence of any tumor at all! Needless to say, she and her family have received the best Christmas present ever. Please send our thanks to Dr. Clark. She has touched another desperately ill person.

JG

Cancer Testimonial #3

I am writing to tell our my story, which is not as dramatic as some, but VERY important to me. I had just begun reading Dr. Clark's "A Cure for All Diseases" because a friend had been diagnosed with cancer. At about that same time, my mammogram showed a highly suspicious growth. My doctor recommended an immediate biopsy, but I decided to give Dr. Clark's protocol a try first. Within 3 weeks, the lump was completely gone, and there has been no trace for 2 yrs. All of this is documented in my medical records.

Just as importantly, by reading Dr. Clark's book, I became aware of things I was using and consuming that contributed to my body's workload. I am a health conscious health care provider, but there were many things I learned about even "health store products"... As a result, I have changed my life, and my health. I continue with Dr. Clark's maintenance protocol, and will do so for the rest of my life. We now make our own soaps, lotions, and shampoos. We use many of Dr. Clark's recipes since she had supplied alternatives to everyday products. I try

to look at everything we use and consume
through Dr. Clark's eyes.

C.C.

Chapter Seventeen
MGN-3

The development of the product known as MGN-3 is relatively new in the field of alternative medicine. But it has exciting promise as a cancer fighter.

There are more than 130 subtypes of white blood cells that make up the immune system. The most important are the T, B, and NK cells. T and B cells are responsible for producing antibodies and chemical messengers (cytokines) that mobilize the immune system for action, while NK cells make up the body's first line of defense. The key to optimum immune system function appears to be not the raw number of NK cells (most people have them in adequate numbers), but the number and activity of the microscopic granules within each NK cell.

By encouraging the development of large numbers of highly active granules within the NK cells, MGN-3 works to "tune up" the immune system while optimizing T, B, and NK cell function.

MGN-3 is manufactured using a patented process that hydrolyzes rice bran with the enzymatic extract of shiitake mushrooms. In published studies, MGN-3 was shown to increase NK cell activity by more than 300%, B cell activity by 250% or greater, and T cell activity by 200% . This is better results than are obtained with any other vitamin, herbal or medicinal mushroom therapies.

Stimulating these immune system cells with MGN-3 gives the immune system the ammunition it needs to keep the entire body in good health.

Sources of MGN-3

1. Better Health International, 2025 Oakland Ave., Indiana PA 15701, Toll Free Tel: 800-772-5568. $39.95

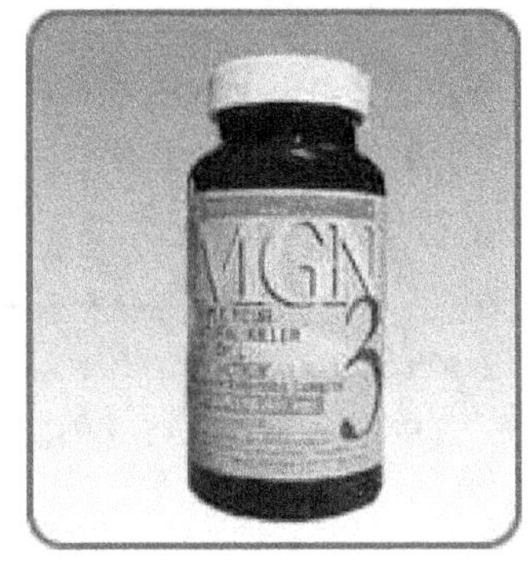

for 50 capsules, 250 mg. each.
2. American Nutrition, 5092 Buttercup Dr.,
   Castle Rock CO 80104, Toll Free Tel:
   800-454-3724. $43.50 for 50 capsules,
   250 mg. each.
3. Brower Enterprises, 102 S Main St.,
   Canton SD 57013, Toll Free Tel" 800-
   373-6076. $49.00 for 50 capsules, 250
   mg. each.

Research Information About MGN-3

Following is excerpted information from several
prominent research reports about MGN-3.
Although a bit technical in nature, these reports
are worth reviewing. Basically, they confirm that
MGN-3 works!

Research Report #1

*Report by: Uyemura, Koichi; Tarchiki, Ken;
Ghoneurn, Mamdooh; Makinodan, Takashi;
Makhijani Nalini; Yamaguchi, Dean of UCLA
Medical School/Greater Los Angeles VA
Healthcare System, Los Angeles CA; Drew
University of Medicine and Science, Los Angeles*

CA and UCLA School of Medicine/Greater Los Angeles VA Healthcare System, Los Angeles CA

There is great interest among health care professionals to explore the value of naturally derived biological response modifiers to enhance immune function. MGN-3 is a biological response modifier that is an arabinoxylan compound which is a polysaccharide containing hemicellulose-b extract of rice bran, modified by enzymes from Shiitake mushrooms reported previously to be a potent immunomodulator. We have previously shown that treatment with MGN-3 had an augmentory effect on natural killer [NK] cell activity in healthy control subjects, in patients with breast cancer, and in patients infected with HIV-1. In these studies, an effect on NK cell activity was noted as early as 4 weeks and did not show hyporesponsiveness with continued treatment for over 12 months, with absence of notable side effects. In the present study, we demonstrate a direct effect of MGN-3 on tumor cell growth and cytokine production. Preliminary results showed that incubation of a breast cancer cell line (MCF-7) with MGN-3 arrested tumor cell growth, whereas control MCF-12A cells grown in a media in the absence of added MGN-3 continued to increase in cell number. Employing flow cytometry procedures, results showed that after 16 hours of treatment of MCF-7 cells with MGN-3 showed a marked stimulation in production of interleukin 10 {IL- 10}. ELISA analyses of the culture media bathing the cells 16 hours after treatment with MGN-3 also showed an increase in IL-10 production, little change in INF-g concentration. However, a marked elevation in Interlukin-12 was also observed at 16 hours. **In conclusion, our findings indicate that MGN-3 acts by not only enhancing the activity of NK cells as previously reported, but also through a direct action on tumor cell production of cytokines.** The production of cytokines such as IL-10 by cancer cells to alter the activity of the immune system is well known. Our findings indicate that the biological response modifier MGN-3 can alter the production and secretion of cytokines such as IL-10 and IL-12 by cancer cells such as MCF-7; and thereby the activity of the immune system. Findings that treatment of cultures of MCF-7 cells with MGN-3 also can arrest cell growth directly may reflect an alternate mechanism of control of tumor cell growth. MGN-3, commercially known as Biobran, was provided by Daiwa Pharmaceuticals Company,

Ltd. Tokyo, Japan. Work in this direction is in progress. Supported in part by VA Medical Research Funds and by funds provided by Daiwa Pharmaceuticals Company, Ltd, Tokyo, Japan

MUSHROOM AMMUNITION
© ALTERNATIVE MEDICINE DIGEST, MAY 1999

Dr. Mamdooh Ghoneum of Charles Drew University of Medicine and Science in Los Angeles compares current cancer treatment to battling terrorists. By bombing a city, you can kill most terrorists, although innocent civilians will also be killed. "Chemotherapy, radiation or surgery are the cancer-equivalents of bombing," he says, "and the beneficial white blood cells in the area are non-terrorist victims." Even after bombing, however, some terrorists may survive, as do those cancer cells that are resistant to the usual therapies. Rather than bombing the city again, however, Dr. Ghoneum advocates sending in Special Forces to locate and eliminate the remaining terrorists one by one.

Dr. Ghoneum's development of a natural supplement called MGN-3 is meant to arm the body's Natural Killer cells to seek and destroy dangerous invaders one by one. The human immune system is comprised of more than 130 subsets of white blood cells. About 15% of them are called Natural Killer (NK) cells. These provide the first line of defense for dealing with any form of invasion to the body. Each cell contains several small granules which act as 'ammunition.' When an NK cell recognizes a cancer cell, for instance, it attaches itself to the cell's outer membrane and injects these granules directly into the interior of the cell. The granules then 'explode,' destroying the cancer cell within five minutes. The killer cell then moves on to other cancer cells and repeats the process. As long as NK cells remain active, the body is able to keep disease under control.

The supplement developed by Dr. Ghoneum, called MGN-3, increases the efficacy of the NK cells. Additionally, it has other immune-boosting effects as well: it increases levels of interferon, a compound produced by the body that inhibits the replication of viruses; it increases the formation of Tumor Necrosis Factors, a group of proteins that help destroy cancer cells; and it increases the activity of T-cells and B-cells. This potent immune system booster is made of the outer shell of rice bran which has been enzymatically treated with extracts from the medicinal Shiitake mushroom. In Japan, mushroom extracts have become the leading prescription treatments for cancer. Dr. Ghoneum's findings have been demonstrated in test-tube experiments as well as seven published studies involving 72 patients. In a study presented to the American Association for Cancer Research, he reported on five patients with breast cancer. Each patient was treated with the same dosage of three grams a day of MGN-3 from a Japanese manufacturer. NK cell activity increased within two weeks and continued to do so as the study progressed. At the end of the six- to eight-month study, two of the patients were in complete remission. In a study reported the following year, 27 patients with various types of cancers including breast, cervical, prostate, leukemia and multiple myeloma were tested for NK cell activity by 51 Chromium release assay before and after only two weeks treatment with MGN-3. NK cell activity increased 154-332% for breast carcinoma, 100-275% in cervical cancer, 174-385% in prostatic cancer, 100-240% in leukemia and 100-537% in multiple myeloma.

One multiple myeloma patient was a 58-year-old
man diagnosed in 1990. He underwent several
months of chemotherapy following his
diagnosis. Although his condition seemed to
stabilize, his blood still showed markers for
multiple myeloma eight months after
chemotherapy. He then began taking MGN-3
and in less than 6 months, follow-up lab work
showed no indication of cancer. Today eight
years after his initial diagnosis, he is the first
patient known to have survived multiple
myeloma, according to Dr. Ghoneum.

Dr. Warren Levin, 66, a holistic physician
practicing in New York City and Ridgefield,
Connecticut, had suffered from an immune
deficiency with an abnormal ratio of helper cells
to suppressor cells since the early '80s. "I tried
herbs, healers, intravenous treatments, all sorts
of stuff. Several years ago, I learned about
glyconutrients — carbohydrate molecules that
play a critically important role in cell-to-cell
communication. I began looking for
glyconutrient sources. All over the world, native

populations were using substances with high glyconutrient content including Aloe Vera, astralagus, echinacea and various mushrooms. At that point, I read an article about MGN-3. I was already taking Coats Aloe Vera Concentrate together with Beta 1-3, D-glucan (Macroforce), Ambrotose, and a thymus preparation called Basic Thymic Protein A as well as the usual vitamins, minerals and antioxidants. I also did intensive mercury detoxification with DMPS. Last fall, I began taking six capsules a day of MGN-3. At the end of December, I sent my blood to the laboratory and when I returned from vacation I found that for the first time in 15 years, every one of my tests had improved well into the middle range of normalcy. That combination of supplements had finally reversed my helper-cell ratio. And normalized my mitogen/allergen responses and NK cell activity."

Dr. Ghoneum's latest study, reported in the International Journal of Immunotherapy, involved 24 patients. Doctors tested NK cell activity in each patient, administered the recommended cancer dosage of 3 grams per day, and tested NK cell activity again after 16 hours, one week, one month and two months. After 16 hours NK cell activity had increased 1.3 to 1.5 times. After one week, activity had increased eightfold. **At the end of two months, NK cells were killing 27 times more cancer cells than prior to taking MGN-3.**

Unlike other forms of cancer treatment, MGN-3 is a totally harmless substance and has no known side effects. In the terrorist analogy, it doesn't kill innocent civilians. David A. Pitts, 73, a real estate salesman in Santa Barbara, California, had undergone chemotherapy for lymphoma treatments with no apparent results. "I had been getting weaker and weaker," he said. After a report on MGN-3, he sent for the supplement and began taking it while he was also placed on a course of intravenous treatment with trioxine, a relatively new drug. "In about three to four weeks on the outside, gosh, I started feeling better," says Pitts. "What really intrigued me was the idea that this supplement could enhance your immune system. When I began, I did a crash program of 14 capsules a day. Now I'm on a preventative program of four a day." At his latest CAT-scan, Pitts was in remission. "The doctor had no explanation of how or why this happened, and there's nothing I can prove. But I'm going to continue taking this for the rest of my life. What's in it is harmless and doesn't interfere with anything else."

Dr. Ghoneum has also used MGN-3 to treat hepatitis B and C and has done in vitro experiments demonstrating its action against HIV. He believes that individuals in "high risk" categories for disease can benefit from using MGN-3 preventively. These include:
• Heavy smokers
• Heavy drinkers
• Individuals, such as artists and house painters, who constantly work with paint
• Those born with immune deficiencies
• Families with a strong history of cancer
• Chemical and refinery workers

Research Report #3

Associate Professor and Chief of Research,
Department of Otolaryngology,
Charles D. Drew University; Research
Associate, Department of Neurobiology,
UCLA School of Medicine

Background:

Although cynicism and disillusionment with the failed "war against cancer" are widespread, I remain very optimistic that we will triumph over this seemingly invincible killer. Given the disappointing results and many drawbacks of cytotoxic therapies, it seems clear that our best hope for a decisive victory against cancer lies in immuno-augmentive therapies, those that enhance the body's innate immune response to cancer cells.

As a research immunologist, I have spent 18 years studying immunomodulating substances — natural compounds derived from mushrooms, herbs, fungi, and bacteria, as well as synthetic drugs like Interleukin-2 and Interferon.

Approximately six years ago, I stumbled across a natural substance that was so promising, so profoundly superior to everything else I had ever evaluated, that I abandoned all other projects, including NIH-funded research, in order to focus entirely on this substance. The product, MGN-3 (an arabinoxylane compound), is a polysaccharide composed of the hemicellose-ß extract of rice bran, modified by enzymes from Shiitake mushrooms. As we have detailed in 7 previously published studies, involving a total of 72 human subjects, the efficacy of MGN-3 equals or surpasses the very best immune-modulating drugs available but, in stark contrast to these, exhibits a complete lack of toxicity. (Copies of complete research papers and data on MGN-3 can be obtained from Lane Labs at 201-236-9090.)

Much of the data regarding MGN-3 has been previously published in technical journals and presented at international research conferences, but the information remains largely unknown to oncologists and other health professionals dealing directly with the cancer patient. The aim of this article is to bring this research to the attention of the practicing clinician, to

summarize what is known about the actions of
MGN-3, and explore its present role in the
treatment of cancer patients.

Anti-viral activity:

In addition to very encouraging results using
MGN-3 in the treatment of malignancies, other
research suggests a promising role for MGN-3
as a therapy for HIV, Hepatitis C, and other viral
infections. MGN-3 has antiviral activity and also
enhances the body's immune response against
virally infected cells. In vitro research shows
that MGN-3 inhibits replication of the HIV virus
without cytotoxicity in a dose-dependent
manner. Human studies suggest that MGN-3
may also be extremely useful in the treatment of
Hepatitis C. In these patients liver enzymes
return to normal levels within 1-8 weeks of
treatment with MGN-3. The results of our
ongoing clinical research into the antiviral
applications of MGN-3 will be the subject of
future reports.

**The role of NK cells in the treatment of
cancer:**

Over 150 different types of white blood cells have been identified and, of these, NK cells are one of the most common, representing up to 15% of total white blood cells. They are important because, unlike other white blood cells, they are able to work more or less independently, not requiring special instructions from the immune system in order to recognize or attack a foreign cell. For this reason, they are often considered to be the body's first line of defense against cancer and viral-infected cells. Circulating through the body by way of the blood and lymph systems, the majority of NK cells present in the body are in a resting state. NK cells become more active in response to immunoregulatory proteins called cytokines. Once activated, the NK cells become quite rapacious in their search-and-destroy activities. Upon encountering a tumor cell, the activated NK cell attaches to the membrane of the cancer cell and injects cytoplasmic granules that quickly dissolve (lyse) the target cell. In less than five minutes, the cancer cell is dead and the NK moves on to its next victim. **A single NK cell can destroy up to 27 cancer cells before it dies. Although quite small in comparison to**

tumor or virus cells, a single NK cell can often bind to two or more cancer cells at once.

The absolute number of NK cells present in the blood gives little indication of the efficiency of immune function. Instead, it is the activity of the NK cells — the avidity with which they recognize and bind to tumor cells — that is important. Most immunomodulators, including MGN-3, do not increase the number or percentage of NK cells, but instead increase their level of activation. NK cell activity can be tested by means of a 4-hour radioactive-Chromium release assay. NK cells are isolated from a blood sample and are incubated in vitro with a fixed number of chromium-labeled tumor cells. After 4 hours, the percentage of tumor cells that have been killed by the NK cells is determined, and this percentage can be used to describe NK cell activity.

In a healthy immuno-competent individual, when NK cell activity is examined at an effector:target ratio of 100:1, we would expect to see NK cell activity ranging from 60-75%. However, in cancer patients, NK cell activity typically ranges from near 0% to 30%. Although it is not entirely clear whether this is a cause or result of the disease process, there is evidence suggesting that low NK cell activity may be a risk factor for malignancy or metastases, as well as a negative prognostic indicator.

Chapter Eighteen

Summary and Conclusion

Please remember that we are researchers, and not physicians. By all means check this information out with your doctor. What is especially attractive about most of these alternative medicine remedies is that they can many times be taken along with traditional medicine protocols. So, in a way, you can perhaps have your cake and eat it too; you can follow the regimen for your cancer that is prescribed by your doctor, and you can take some of these alternative therapies also. Ask your doctor about it.

There are too many alternative holistic therapies mentioned in this book to take all at once. So you may wish to rely on your own inner guidance and select a few to try out. Generally, most people report that only a few weeks are needed in order to tell if they are being helped. You should get some sort of indication that these therapies are working. It may be a greater sense of well-being, or signs of detoxification, or signs of lessened cancer activity. Trust your inner senses and guidance.

Bonus Addendum!

Saving the Best for the Last

Our Amazing Healing Discovery

In 2021 I made my most important healing discovery. I wish to share it with you. So here goes.

I began to study artificial intelligence. In reading up on the QFS (quantum financial system) that was just beginning to emerge in the banking system, I found some intriguing and hard-to-believe information. There was plenty of

information available about what the QFS would
do for mankind (better, faster banking, more
honest and dependable system, etc.) there was
little or no information about how it worked.

I have a personal rule; if I don't understand it, I
avoid it. So I jumped into a quick study to see if
I could understand it, since it seemed so
important to the future of mankind.

Briefly, what I discovered is that as computers
got more and more sophisticated, and faster and
faster, and more "intelligent", scientists were
reaching the point where they had learned how
to interface computers with the human mind. I
will not go any further in this explanation,
because, frankly, it get freaky and hard-to-
believe if you go any deeper.

As I was working my way through all of this, I
got some advice in meditation. My spirit guides
advised me not to fret because mankind had
already been using this technology for a
thousand years. They then mentioned the Holy
Water used by the Catholic Church.

Years ago, when I practiced Radionics healing
extensively, I had, yes, learned that Holy Water

does have special healing power. I had actually bought some Holy Water online, placed it in test tube, and had used it as a "reagent" to speed up certain healing processes. In other words, when I added the vibrational qualities of the Holy Water to the vibrations that were being sent to a person's affliction, the healing process was improved. So I knew that Holy Water was special.

I next went to the Internet to learn more about Holy water. Here is how it is made; a group of Priests fill a church fountain or other container with water and then they pray over it. They, in essence, bless the water. Then it becomes Holy Water. Pretty simple.

There are 3 prayers that they may use for this process. All are basically the same. Here is one of them:

"Blessed are you, Lord, all-powerful God, who in Christ, the living water of salvation, blessed and transformed us. Grant that when we are sprinkled with this water or make use of it, we will be refreshed inwardly by the power of the Holy Spirit and continue to walk in the new life we received at Baptism."

I was surprised that the simplicity of this prayer. Basically, all it does is commit the water to the wonderful power of God.

Then things got really wonderful and special. This is hard to explain, but I will try my best to explain it to you.
I was told that the water being blessed and prayed over was capable of assisting mankind much more. But it had to be instructed by God to do so. Then the water would directly (in the case of illness), attack and remove the illness. Or in case of emotional distress, remove the harmful emotions and restore the body to happiness and balance.

Basically, this process changes the water in your body from a passive status to a status where it becomes an active healing agent. It was emphatically stressed that, unless the water as asked by God to do this, it would not work.

Where an understanding of Artificial Intelligence comes in

If you ponder on this for a while, as I have done, things become more clear. Artificial Intelligence involves establishing a link with the human mind and a non-human object (the computer). This link goes through God. God somehow allows this link (information) to be passed on to other mechanisms in God's realm, and the work is done. Not a great explanation, but is the best that I can offer, given my own limitations.

Well, the same basic thing happens with Holy Water. I have explained this in other sections of my book "On Stormy Seas". The written works of Viktor Shauberger and Masaru Emoto also delve sufficiently to explain water's ability to carry conscience and intelligence.

Thus when the Priests pray over the water, they impart a request that God bless the water with their message. God does this, and from then on the water has special curative powers. The water then later passes this curative power on to you.

So my Spirit Guides are right. The enlightenment of our knowledge of artificial intelligence does lead us right back to the knowledge of Holy Water that has been known for a thousand years. Interesting.

Where are we going with this?

I have to be careful here, as I do not wish to inadvertently reveal anything that I am not supposed to reveal.

What my Spiritual Advisors have told me is to take the basic prayer to bless Holy Water and "soup it up" by asking the water to do extra things, which it will most probably be happy to do for you and God. Remember always that God is approving everything, so you cannot inadvertently ask for anything that goes against God's will. Should you accidently do so, it is simple. God will not grant your request.

So, my first chance to use this knowledge came when two of my beloved Essiac employees got sick from taking Covid vaccinations shots. They drank this water. They immediately got better. I have also been using this knowledge to improve my own health and well as helping my wife deal with some health issues. It is working for us. I am going to list here several of the requests that we have been using.

Dear God, Please instruct this water to remove all harmful substances from my body. Please remove all illness and disease from my body. Please remove all harm from the Covid and the Covid vaccinations. Thank you. We love you.	Dear God, Please instruct the water in my body to restore my energy levels to that of a 35 year-old person. Thank you and I love you.
Dear God, Please instruct this water to heal And cure the swelling in my feet And legs. Thank you. I love you.	Dear God, Please instruct this water to remove the excess and unhealthy fat from my body And restore my body shape to a healthy Condition. I love you. Thank you.
Dear God, Please instruct the water to	Dear God, Please instruct the water to

remove all arthritis from my body. Remove all bone joint deposits. Thank you and I love you.	remove all diabetes from my body. Remove all acidity from my pancreas. Thank you and I love you.

Here is the system that I use; I use a credit card sized energy plate. I buy mine at purpleplates.com. These aluminum plates are imbued with life force energy. I have used them successfully for many years for other healing purposes. I then perform a consecration ritual where I pass the message for my healing to the energy plate, all the while asking God to approve everything. I then print the prayer request, cut it out, ask God to bless it (through a prayer) and tape it to the energy plate. I cover everything in plastic. I then take this energy plate and tape it or fasten it to the water pipe feeding the faucet where I draw my drinking and cooking water. Sometimes, depending on the complexity of the house water piping system, I just fasten the plate to the cold water line that feeds the house (usually near the water heater).

Thus the blessed message is passed on to the water that I drink. The water does the rest. Some people prefer to carry the energy plate in their pocket. Either method works. After a while you may get your own inspiration on various ways to use this information. Just be sure to get God's permission.

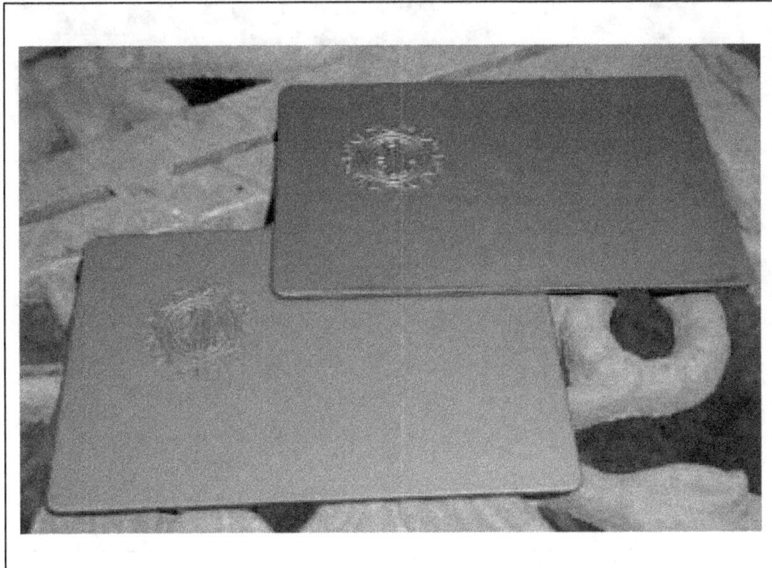

Energy plates (credit card size)

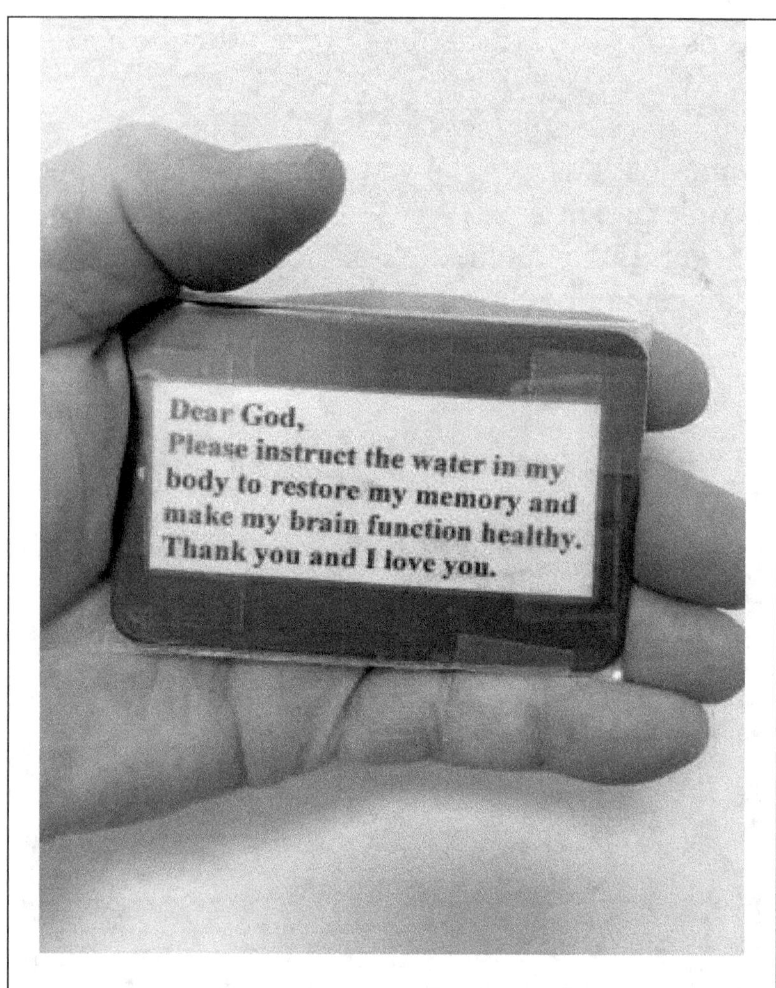

The finished product. Fasten to your water pipes.

ADDENDUMS

Special Bonus Section
Additional Information for our Inquisitive Readers
Contains some controversial views, so Proceed at your own Risk!

Do you know anyone who has skin cancer? If so, you may wish to show them this information. This inexpensive cream really works!

Our "Super Dooper" Skin Cancer Salve

There are two ingredients in our "Super Dooper" skin cancer salve:

Hydrogen Peroxide.
The main ingredient is liquid hydrogen peroxide. It is not just any-old drug store variety of peroxide. It is a special kind of hydrogen peroxide that is labeled **"35% Food Grade Hydrogen Peroxide"**.
This special peroxide can be found at many health food stores, or it can be bought online. The last 16 oz. bottle that I bought cost me about $20.00. It will last me about 6 months.

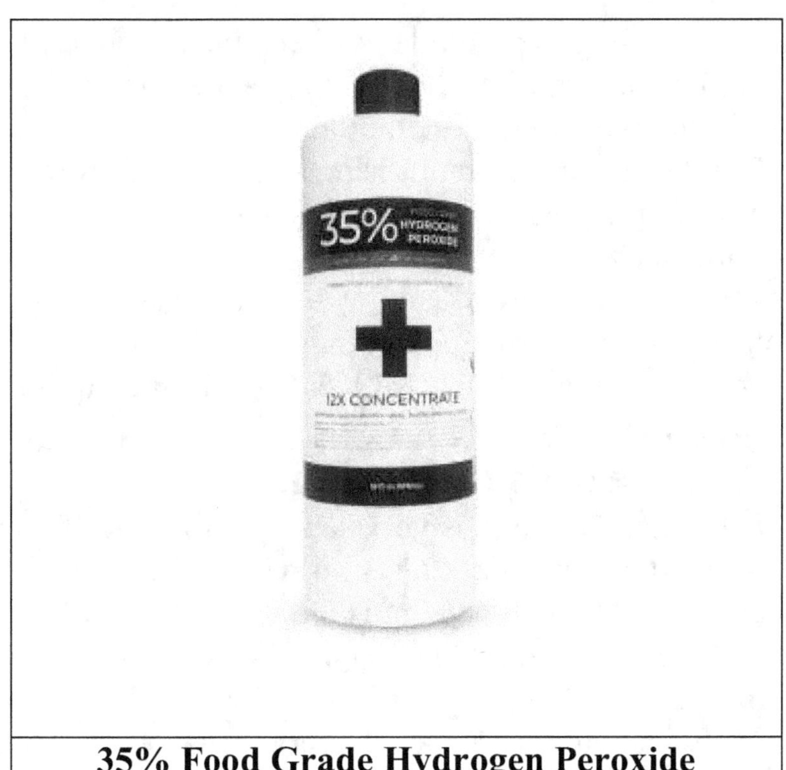

35% Food Grade Hydrogen Peroxide

How it works.

The chemical expression for hydrogen peroxide is H_2O_2. When the hydrogen peroxide is placed on your skin, it transfers to H_2O (water) and O (a free molecule of oxygen). This free molecule of oxygen is very reactive. It wants to quickly bond with something else.

If the hydrogen peroxide has been placed on a malignant tumor (such as a skin cancer tumor) it will quickly bond with the tumor.

But the cancerous tumor is anaerobic; it cannot exist in the presence of oxygen. Thus it immediately dies.

And that, dear friend is how it works. It works fast. It is simple to apply. And, in my many years of using this salve, I have never failed to see it work properly.

A few words of caution.

Hydrogen peroxide is very sensitive to light. If it is not stored in a dark place, it will deteriorate quickly. It should be kept is a light- proof bottle, and the bottle should be stored in a cool, dark place.

Also, it should be replaced every year-or-so. Age will reduce its strength.

Aloe Vera Gel.

The other ingredient is aloe vera gel.

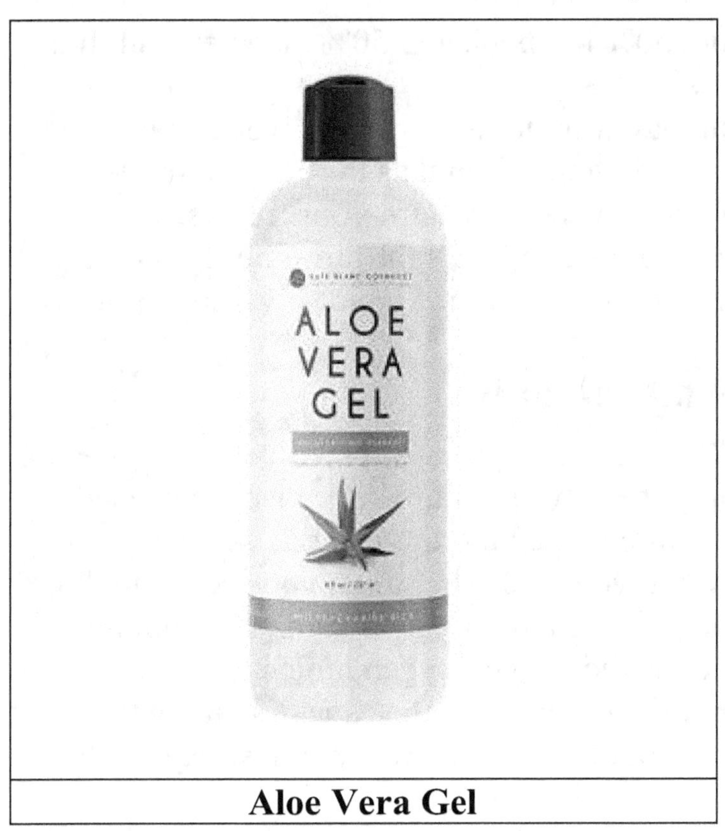

Aloe Vera Gel

This is easier to obtain. You can find it at almost any drug store, grocery store, or health food store. A 16 oz. bottle or jar costs me about $16.00.

Making the Salve:

Making the salve is incredibly easy. Just mix up the amount that you will need. Make the ration

about 50% peroxide and 50% aloe vera gel. It is
that simple.
You may want to use a plastic, wood or metal
spoon for your mixing, as the 35% peroxide is
very strong and may burn your fingers.
Store your salve in a light-proof bottle and keep
in in a dark place (a refrigerator works fine).

Using the Salve:

Apply the salve to your skin cancer as needed.
The more you apply, the faster it will act.
If, when you apply the salve, you see a bubbling
action, this is a really good sign. The bubbling
action is the active oxygen molecule in the
peroxide mixing with the cancerous growth.
You should see results within a few days.

Note: This information is extracted from the
book **"The Skin Cancer Information
Handbook"** by Michael D. Miller.

Another Bonus Chapter!

Explaining Where We Came From, and Where Sacred Geometry Came From: A Fable Story

I am presenting the following information as a fable. Why a fable? Because I cannot prove to you that it is true. But, like many fables, some people believe that it is true. Including me. This fable is put together from 40 years of reading, meditation, studies, and pondering. So I am offering it to you for your amusement/consideration.

By virtue of your open-mindedness that you have shown in reading this book, I am assuming that some of you may appreciate this information. It is offered to you in the spirit of friendship and appreciation for reading my book. Let's "fable" onward.

About Sacred Geometry: In order to explain where it is that sacred geometry and the concepts and knowledge of how to harness the powers of sacred geometry came from, we first have to delve into the matter of how mankind was created.

Most of our knowledge here is offered to us from the bible. But the bible was written two thousand years ago, during a time when most people were illiterate and uneducated. So the written stories in the bible of our creation may have served well two thousand years ago. But today we seek better and more complete knowledge.

Thus it is that stories such as this are written.

Zachariah Sitchin

As a quick introduction, here is how Wikipedia explains this man:

Zechariah Sitchin (July 11, 1920 – October 9, 2010)[1] was an author of a number of books proposing an explanation for human origins involving ancient astronauts. Sitchin attributed the creation of the ancient Sumerian culture to the Anunnaki, which he stated was a race of extraterrestrials from a planet beyond Neptune called Nibiru. He asserted

Many years ago I began to read the books written by this famous anthropologist Zachariah Sitchin. He was said to be the only person who could read the ancient Sumerian hieroglyphic clay tablets and scrolls.

His writing were different, they were provocative. Few experts agreed with him. But he stated some very important things, things that made sense. Things that meshed with other facts of the scientific community.

As I checked him out, I found that he really was the only scientist in the world who could read the ancient Sumerian hieroglyphics. These ancient clay tablets were from antiquity. And Mr. Sitchin drew much of his information from them. A prolific writer, he wrote about 12 books, all based on information from analysis of the Sumerian clay tablets. He told the creation of man story from a different perspective, a different viewpoint. And his stories were interesting! So I, over the years, read many of his books.

Then I hit pay dirt. Just before he retired, he published the book **"The Lost Book of Enki"**. It told the story of mankind's creation, as seen through the eyes of several of the ancient Alien beings that had inhabited earth. They had created mankind to use as a slave race to help them mine the abundant gold deposits that they found on earth.

His story really made sense to me. His story, as always, was based on information that he had gleaned from the ancient Sumerian hieroglyphics. It was consistent with the bible, and all known information about our creation. Mr. Sitchin has since passed away. But his information made a big impression on me, and gave me a newly expanded knowledge about how we were created.

Then a fascinating guy by the name of Clif High also published a report about the creation of mankind. It meshed perfectly with the material presented by Zachariah Sitchin. Plus it gave an interesting insight into how the Egyptian

Mystery Schools were created, and where the information taught in the Egyptian Mystery Schools came from.

What was Zachariah Sitchin's Information about Creation? Here, in a nutshell, is what Mr. Sitchin told us in his book *The Lost Book of Enki*: A group of Aliens known as the Anunnaki came to earth eons ago. They were searching for gold, a mineral scarce on their own planet. They found plenty of gold on earth. They were not a race of beings that were used to doing labor. Therefore they attempted to mine gold using the local beings that they found on earth. This did not work. The local people were also not good workers. They set about to clone a new race of beings who would be good workers (miners). They developed a cloned being that was made up of beings from the planet Sirius, with strands of DNA added to "dumb them down" to make them controllable workers. The added strands (2 strands) of DNA were from a reptilian source.

1.

This new cloned being was a successful
venture. Gold mining progressed.

2.

The new beings multiplied and became
numerous.

3.

Eventually the Anunnaki decided to return
to their home, the planet Niburu.
They arranged for the Great Flood that
would destroy their cloned worker society.
Some enlightened Anunnaki objected to
the destruction of the worker society, they
interfered, and thus some of mankind
survived the deluge.And thus we were
created to eventually multiply and cover
the earth.

My interesting observation: The Sirians were a
pure race of people, very spiritual and honest.
When the cloners added two strands of reptilian
DNA to the Sirian body, they created good
workers for their mines. But they also had
introduced into our being a capacity for evil that
the Sirians did not have.

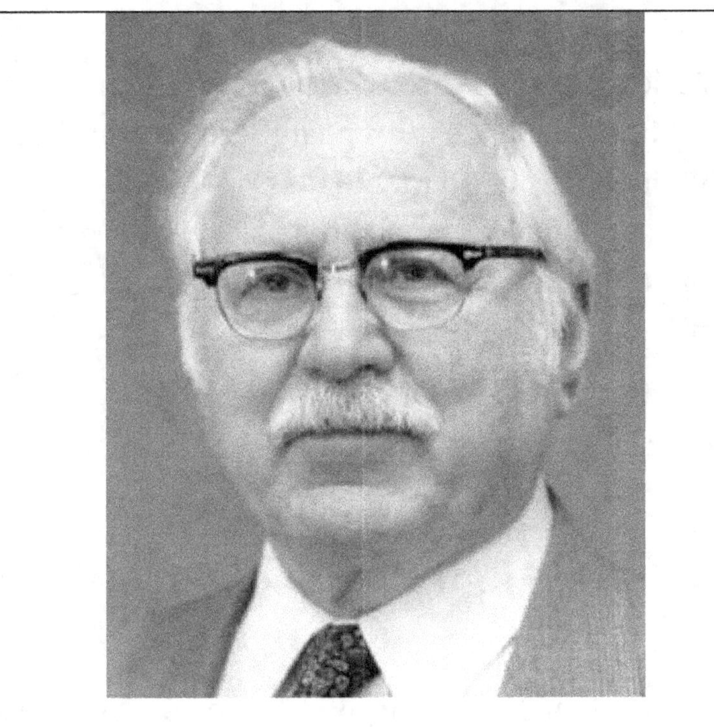

Zachariah Sitchin

I find this information consistent with many writing that discuss God and his plan for mankind. Many see that God's plan is for us to overcome this tendency toward evil that was bred into mankind. When we have finally overcome this handicap, we will all joyfully return to be with God forever. We will be experienced "warriors" who have fought the good fight and have triumphantly returned to the God that loves us so much!

Anyway, let us now look at the story of mankind's creation as told by my esteemed guru Clif High.

Clif High's story of Creation

About Clif High: For over 14 years I have been a fan of Clif High. He first made a name for himself by developing a method for extracting predictions from the language patterns of mankind. He was hired by major corporations to utilize his information. He eventually retired to the woods of Washington state, where he pumps out a very interesting newsletter.

I have found his information sincere and truthful.

An article written by him follows:

<u>This colony, Earth.</u>
We've been invaded by Space Aliens!

This Colony, Earth.

We've been invaded by Space Aliens

Six thousand years ago, more or less, Earth was invaded by Space Aliens.

They came down all around the planet, in the lands just north of the Tropic of Cancer. The Space Alien invasion arrived in a small, but heavily armed, force, with the clear intent to conquer and colonize Earth.

They landed in Yucatan Peninsula. They landed in Macedonia, Sumer, India, China, and Japan, and elsewhere.

From these bases, their superior technology which included over 40 different types of flying war machines, they easily conquered the hunter-gatherer tribes inhabiting the area.

In each area thus conquered, the local tribes provided the name for the Space Aliens in their own language. Thus we know the Colonists as the Elohim, the Devas, the Theoae, the Anunnaki, the Shin, and in all cases, in all languages those names became synonymous with 'gods'.

Once the local tribes were conquered, the Space Aliens conscripted their local human population to go forth, and conquer other, more distant tribes of humans. They did so, with the occasional assistance of the Space Alien 'lords'.

As the combat local to the landing sites faded away, the Space Alien overlords set about building vast complexes on the conquered territory. These were called GANS in their language, which our religious texts today, translate as 'gardens'.

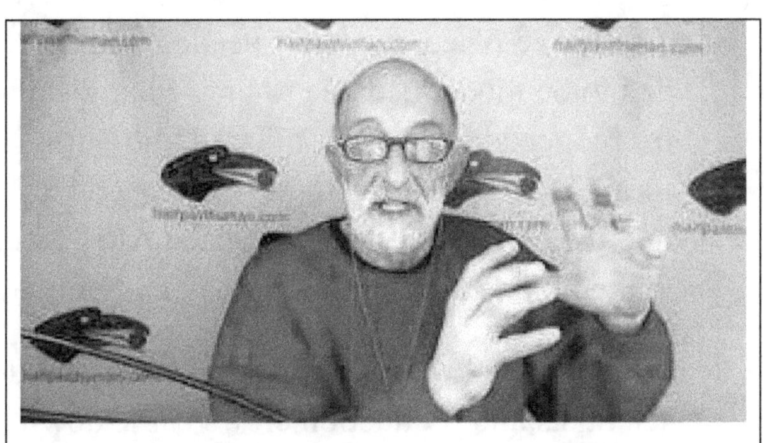

Clif High, Internet Guru, developer of "Predictive Linguistics"

These GANS were the Space Alien's genetic material production laboratories. These GANS had 'energy shields' which prevented non-authorized access by the local populations of humans. It is thought now that the GANS enclosed several hundreds of square kilometers of area, rising several thousands of feet. These energy shields also provided both air, and light filtration.

The Space Alien overlords needed both. The light had to be moderated due to their biological needs for reduced levels of cosmic radiation of all forms. The air needed to be sterilized as it flowed into the GANS because the Space Aliens were vulnerable to earth bacteria to an extreme level.

As the GANS were stabilized, the Space Alien scientists and production crews came down to Colony Earth, and set to work. Their goal was to create a smart-enough, but not too smart, slave species.

The work in the GANS continued for approximately 2000 years.

It was difficult work, building an effective slave species from the local genetic base merged with part of the genetic material of the Space Alien Colonists. There were many wrong choices made, and species were created, then destroyed when they did not meet specifications. Some, including the Giants, escaped the GANS to roam about the land, but as these beings were engineered, and not native to this environment, they failed to thrive, all eventually succumbing to adverse conditions.

About 4000 years ago, a certain level of success in the engineering of the Colonists was achieved with the creation of the first of the 'white people'. Variously, the Space Aliens had already, from the native brown humans, created Black, Yellow, Red, and then finally White people.

It was difficult work, and it would seem that the Space Alien Colonists stopped their genetic engineering with the creation of the white people. It is not known if this was due to their goal being achieved, or if external, adverse circumstances altered the direction of the Space Alien overlords' efforts.

Shortly after their successful engineering of their slave species, the Space Alien Colonists left earth.

We don't know, for sure, why they left.

There are hints, in our ancient literature, that rising cosmic radiation levels created conditions on Earth that greatly increased the risk to the Space Alien Colonists in the form of bacterial infection. The Space Alien overloads were very long lived, especially when protected by the filtration of the energy shields around the GANS. It is thought that they lived many thousands of years, perhaps, in a protected environment, into the 10's of thousands of years. Though the Colonists were protected, and long lived, they were acutely afraid of death.

Out in the wild, that is, in the unprotected areas of Colony Earth, the Space Alien Colonists had need of extraordinary precautions to avoid bacterial infections of which, even minor ones were rapidly fatal.

About 4000 years ago, conditions changed here on Earth for the Colonists, and they left. The leaving was a mass exodus that was completed in a remarkably short period of time.

It is speculated that there was some level of failure of the GANS energy shields that prompted the Space Alien Colonists to flee.

The failure, and removal of the GANS structures allowed the engineered slave species the freedom to walk the Earth. As an engineered species, and non-native to this environment, the created Humans struggled to survive, though, they were successful.

It greatly aided the newly liberated slave species that the food stock animals and plants built by the Colonists to feed their slaves were very hardy within the Earth's biosphere, spreading across the lands.

When the Space Alien Colonists left Earth, the managerial class of slaves, who were the go-between for the Space Aliens in their interaction with their created slave species, moved in to fill the power vacuum.

At that time, there was a concerted effort on the part of the managerial class of slaves to claim the power that had been held by the Space Alien Colonists.

The managers declared themselves a 'priest'

class, moved the now absent Space Alien
Overlords from a status of physical beings into a
category of 'transcendent omnipotent invisible
gods', and declared that they, the priests, were the
only ones with 'authority', both here on Earth,
over other members of the slave species, as well
as with the intercession process of
communication with the Space Alien overlords.

It was a sweet gig for the priest class. Too good,
too soft & cushy of a position, to easily surrender.
Thus the many ills associated with the
implementation of religion can be seen to arise
from these circumstances.

As also may be inferred, thus arose the human
practice of Colonization, of War, as we practice
it, of Law as it pertains to interactions between
ourselves, and many, many other attributes of our
lives here, in this resulting, now.

Civilization, as we know it now, is not a human
invention. It was impressed upon the engineered
descendants of the original hunter-gatherer tribes
by the invading Colonists, both by pressure of

force, and by cultural mimicry of the newly formed humans adopting the superior ways of the Space Alien Colonists over the tribal forms of their precedents who provided the base biological source for their genetics.

There have been other civilizations here on Earth. They existed prior to the coming of the Space Alien Colonists.

There have been other, modern humans, here on Earth, who built those civilizations. We are separated from them by the Great Ice Age.

Our antecedents, those hunter-gatherer tribes, were themselves a remnant of the previous ages of Humans, here on Earth. If it had not been for the impact of the Great Ice upon the previous Age of Man here on Earth, the Space Alien Colonists might not have had such an easy time of it with our ancestors.

Though the priest class will maintain that the Space Alien Colonists 'created' modern humans in their GANS laboratories, do not be deceived.

The Space Aliens are not gods, they are tinkerers. They made small tweaks in humanity, they did not create us. Their goal was to make us just-smart-enough, and docile.

It did not quite work. Humans are far smarter than the Colonists wanted, and not close enough to docile to be able to be controlled, as our priest class is constantly complaining. Perhaps this contributed to the Exodus. Maybe, when we get our species collective ass out into space, and we find these Space Alien Colonists, we can ask them.
Clif High

My Summary and Conclusions about the Anunnaki and our knowledge of Sacred Geometry

The Anunnaki had created their "worker race" who would do their mining for them on earth. In the process of organizing this work force, it was necessary to have some of these workers be supervisors in order to direct the rest of the workers.

 Thus it was, in the thousands of years that followed, a separate level or "Order of Supervisors" was established. They were ranked as superior to the worker force, but were, of course, lower than the lowest Anunnaki supervisors.

Then, eventually, the decision to abandon earth had been made. Enki and his friends had taken steps to insure that some of their "worker force" had survived the deluge that was set upon the earth to destroy the workers (the legend of Noah and his ark?). Then the Anunnaki left earth, leaving the surviving workers to fend for themselves. Some of these surviving workers were of the Supervisor class.

These surviving Survivor class workers had, though their closer contact with the Anunnaki, learned much of the Anunnaki wisdom and knowledge. Because the Supervisors had superior knowledge and information, it was easy for them to establish themselves as the new ruling class. This morphed into them becoming the Religious or Priestly Class who ruled over the more-ordinary masses.

Among this knowledge of the Priestly Class was knowledge of the principles of sacred geometry, and how the Anunnaki had utilized this knowledge to enhance their lives and work.

As Priestly classes tend to do, they did not share their esoteric knowledge with the masses. They hoarded this information in order to increase their power over the masses. Thus it was, that with time, arcane knowledge of things such as sacred geometry, was only known by a special group of the Priestly Class (I will hereinafter refer to them as the "Priests").

With this as a background, mankind began his sojourn on earth.

God took advantage of this situation. He set up a plan to enrich the knowledge and wisdom of select angels.

God sent these angels to live on the earth as men, and to begin the long and difficult path to attaining enlightenment. They had to overcome the challenges offered here on earth. These challenges were due to the reptilian strands in our bodies that gave us a capacity for evil. When we have overcome the challenges that are found here on earth (i.e., having overcome our capacity for evil), we will once again be reunited with God. This is God's plan for us. It is a great plan. When we have won our struggle and have returned to God we will be wiser and more enlightened. We will, in short, be more godlike.

His love for us, and our love for Him, will be increased immensely. We will be Super Angels. This is his gift to us. Yes, it is a great plan. For thousands of years the powers of sacred geometry existed, but most of mankind didn't know about it. So as we now progress onward, knowledge of things such as sacred geometry is coming to us. It comes in bits and pieces, but it comes. This perhaps means that it is time for us to relearn this ancient knowledge. Perhaps that is why you are reading this book.

Why the World Is the Way it is

(This writing is offered as part of the Bonus Section to the book. It is very political in nature. If it offends you in any way, I apologize. Please, if you are offended, do not read any further!)

{**Author Comment**: I think that it is okay to include this extra chapter in the book. I believe that Franklin Delano Roosevelt was part of the elite members of our society who supported and were benefitted by the group that we today refer to as the "One World Order" crowd; OWO". In other words, FDR could murder 50,000 Americans and get away with it because he was part of this elitist group. Their control over the media gave them awesome power to influence the American people. This article explains how this all happened.

In this bonus chapter I attempt to explain how the elite became so powerful. So powerful, in effect, that a man like FDR, of the political elite, could get away with openly condemning 50,000 Americans to death and destruction, in a wanton act of petty jealousy and deceit. And the public, manipulated by the media, said nothing. It also helps to explain the power wielded by the military-industrial establishment (also part of the OWO) so that they could get MacArthur fired in order to get their bigger war in Korea that they sought. (again, refer to the Fletcher Prouty book mentioned above).}

Dear Reader,

For many years now I have suffered silently as I have watched well-meaning but mis-guided American patriots expound their ideas and beliefs about what is wrong with the world. Quite frankly, these guys are mostly wrong. They mean well, but they simply don't know who the bad guys are.

My experiences in Vietnam taught me that we are not told the truth. So I set about to find the truth. After many years of research, I finally think that I know who the bad guys are. So I am now speaking up. The attached article explains all this. Many of you will have problems accepting this information, basically because it will probably conflict with many of your long-held belief systems. I understand this because I also had to surmount this obstacle on my way to learning the truth.

History of the Banking World: After the violence of the French Revolution in the 1700s, a period of political and public instability reigned in France. Then an obscure army officer, Napoleon Bonaparte, rose to prominence and took over the country. Napoleon's greatest gift

was as a military leader, so he launched France on a series of military campaigns. Up to then, military campaigns had been financed simply; the victor stole the wealth of the conquered and took it home with them. But the old way of doing things did not work for Napoleon because he overloaded the system with his constant war campaigns. So a group of enterprising bankers, led by the Rothschild ("red shield") families, offered for their banks to finance Napoleon's wars. [Note: The Rothschild family was from the Khazar nation, a tribe from Russia. Their warlike nature led the czar to banish them from Russia. They had just settled in Europe and embraced the Jewish religion, although they had no historic Jewish roots. Actually, the actual Jewish people have suffered more at the hands of the Rothschild One World Order than any other group on the planet.]
Napoleon readily agreed to have them finance his wars. Over the ensuing years, Napoleon's constant warfare made the French bankers very rich. But, how did the Rothschild bankers get the money to finance Napoleon's expensive wars? Here is how it was done: Initially people paid for things with money, most of which was gold or silver. But big business transactions were complicated by the difficulty of transporting and

storing when many tons of gold and silver were required. So someone invented a simpler way. They simply issued a warehouse receipt to the owners of the gold and silver that these people owned, and the people used the warehouse receipt to pay in lieu of the actual gold and silver. This was a big improvement in the way things were done. But the bankers noted that people seldom ever returned to collect the gold and silver from the banker's vaults. They just kept trading the warehouse receipts back and forth. So the clever, if also a bit unscrupulous, bankers began to issue "duplicate" receipts to borrowers. This made each of these transactions 100% profit for the bankers, because when the new loan was paid off, all 100% of the principal of the funds went into the banker's pockets, plus the interest. Most of Napoleon's wars were financed with such "fiat" money.

So Napoleon's wars were financed with this "made-up" money, and given Napoleon's power, no one questioned it. This was the birth of fiat banking.

Within a generation, the Rothschild banking families had become incredibly rich. They then used this newfound wealth to place younger members of the banking families into all of the power centers of the European countries. They eventually controlled governments, the banks, the churches, the militaries, etc. In short, they became the most important and powerful group in Europe. They then gained control of all the major banks, replacing the legitimate currencies with their "fiat" money, which was backed by nothing but air.

Their wealth and power had also led to excesses. Many of the Europeans who fled to the newly discovered America fled to escape the abuses of the powerful and despotic European Rothschild banking empires.

For instance, when one studies the life and trials of Andrew Jackson in America, it is discovered that he spent most of his life trying to thwart the inroads that the European bankers were making to gain control of our banking system so that they could institute their fiat money banking system that tended to rob the public of its wealth and prosperity.

Patriots such as Andrew Jackson kept the European bankers at bay. Then, in 1913, in a carefully planned event, they secretly got passed the Federal Reserve Act. This gave them ownership of the American currency. They replaced the American dollar (which was worth one dollar in gold) with the Federal Reserve note (which was backed by nothing).

If this does not seem possible, you may read the book "*The Creature from Jekyll Island*" by G. Edward Griffin which details this event.

In the Political World: While the banking side of the Rothschild Empire was exploiting the banking systems of Europe, other branches of the family had established themselves in the religious and intellectual establishments of Europe. This included the Templar Knight movement that had evolved into the Freemason movement.

One aspect of the Freemason beliefs was to establish a more perfect world, and this involved a long-term plan to gradually replace corrupt government and religious movements that exploited the people with a more perfect leadership in terms of equality and justice, a form of world leadership that was truly just and honest. One has to admire their tremendous piety and honor and idealism to tackle such a formidable objective.

The Freemason also played a prominent part in establishing our form of government, emphasizing freedom and equality for all.

When the ruling members of the Rothschild Empire found out that there was a movement afoot to replace all of the separate governments of the world with a new order that would control

all of the world, they decided to replicate this movement. After all, if someone was going to run the world, it should be them because they controlled most of the wealth of the world. **Thus was born the "One World Order" Movement**: It is controlled, financed and directed by the Rothschild Empire. In the ensuing 250-some years, they have used their ability to issue money as needed (free to them), to entrench their movement very deeply into most aspects of our lives. They exert control over our media, Hollywood, the medical establishments, the politicians in Washington DC, our political parties, the church, and most of the major industries in the United States.
If you are having problems digesting this information, you are not alone. Most of us have experienced this. The massiveness of the evil and corruption is so great that it is hard for our human minds to process this information. But as you will find if you dig deeper, this information is true.
Mystical Aspects: When the Rothschild One World Order movement began, they adopted and copied much of the knowledge that the Templar Knights had brought back to Europe at the end of the Crusades (about the year 1300). This included much of the knowledge and wisdom of

the Egyptian Mystery Schools. For some 300 years the Templar Knights had studied the wisdom and knowledge of the Egyptian ancient empire. They were thoroughly indoctrinated with this ancient knowledge which included ancient rituals. Unfortunately some of these ancient rituals involved prayers and rituals that could be used toward the "dark side" of life. Thus it was that the Rothschild agents learned of some ancient rituals that involved using black magic to control and affect the behavior of others. The Rothschild (One World Order) agents incorporated some of these rituals into their practices, since they were consistent with the One World Order goal of controlling and domination over other peoples. As the OWO (One World Order) movement was embedding itself into the fabric of European society and life, they found it helpful to use some of these rituals to rather forcefully gain the loyalty and compliance of leaders and spokesmen of European society.

Here is how it was done. A young person was rising quickly up the OWO chain of promotion. Then he was presented with a special "opportunity" to participate in some secret ritual. It was widely accepted that, were he to decline, he would never advance any further. So he

usually accepted the invitation. What he did not
know is that this ritual would involve doing
something despicable (by normal standards). So,
under the great pressure of the moment, he
complied. But what he had done was
compromise himself so the OWO people now
had information that could forevermore be used
to blackmail or control him.

Now the OWO people had an obedient servant
who had to do their bidding for the rest of his
life.

So, you ask, what sort of despicable behavior
was involved? Some consisted of deviant sexual
behavior, sometimes with small children. Other
times, it involved human sacrifice. We do not
wish to overstate these matters. But for you to
understand the depth and difficulty of opposing
these OWO forces that are attempting to
destabilize our country, you have to know this.
We are facing great evil.

How does this affect us? As the OWO
movement established itself deeper and deeper
into the Fabric of American society, the above
described practices were used in America to also
draw into and control all of the OWO people
who had been recruited. It has gotten so bad that
US military forces who are loyal to the
Constitution and the country have actually

invaded and liberated underground centers where these dark practices were centered.

We believe that some of these truths will be revealed to the American public in the upcoming years. The shock of all this will be difficult for the American public to accept or understand.

The OWO Timetable: Documents have been found that state that the original OWO goal was to complete their conquest of the world by the year 2000. This seems to be tied to ancient Egyptian knowledge that relates to the dimensions and other information gleaned from the Great Pyramid at Giza. I have seen a photo of George Bush Sr. holding a small replica of the Great Pyramid in his hand and stating "We are almost on schedule".

Well, as we now know, they are now behind schedule. And there is great opposition to their movement. The BRICS Alliance seems to exist as a major deterrence to their plans for conquest. The American media ignores the BRIC existence, but these 149 countries that have banded together are a formidable opponent. Russia, as a member of the BRICS Alliance, is a major leader.

Where does the USA fit into all this? The OWO crowd has poured billions of dollars of fake money into our country for many years. Thus it is that they control all the media, most of the politicians, and most of our industry. We do not get the truth from our media; we get the narratives that the OWO wants us to get. Our government no longer represents the people, it now represents the narratives pushed by the OWO, cleverly pitched to convince us that it is actually doing what is best for us.

Why Have I Done This: Why have I opened up myself to the criticism and grief that I will get for writing this article? It is because I am frustrated. I am frustrated because I see that 99% of the American public is being hoodwinked. 99% of the American public does not even know who the enemy is.

The real enemy is the One World Order.

Take the situation in the Ukraine. 99% of us believe that Russia is the bad guy. Americans are ready to go over there and die to kill those damned Russians. Wow! Have the OWO guys done a good job or what? Russia is not the bad guy. The OWO is the bad guy. They overthrew the legitimate government of the Ukraine in 2014 (using $5 Billion of US State Department money) and installed a pro-Nazi government. They have then used this pro-Nazi government to provoke and antagonize the next-door Russians. Remember that twenty million

Russians died in WWII fighting the nazi invasion. Anti-nazi sentiment in Russia still runs deep!

Also, remember the Russian Missile Crisis of 1962? We were ready to start WWIII because the Russians legally and openly installed missile in Cuba, 90 miles from our shores. Now we do not seem to understand why our installing nazi-backed missiles and US military on Russia's border is a problem? But with our media spoon-feeding us OWO misinformation, we are being led down the primrose path. Have we forgotten the Monroe Doctrine?

What is the OWO trying to accomplish? I can only guess. But a WWIII scenario will probably destroy a great part of our country, weaken us, and allow the OWO people to take over. If they gain control of the USA, the rest of the world will quickly follow.

If they gain control of Russia, they will be able to take over the Russian banks and install their system of fiat money to ruin and control Russia. They will then control all of the major banking centers of the western world. They will also be able to more easily thwart the efforts of the BRICS alliance, since Russia is one of their leaders.

Further Comments: There is an excellent book that gives good detail about much of this, written by a retired US military intelligence officer, Colonel Fletcher Prouty.
The book is "*JFK, Vietnam, and the Plot to Assassinate John F. Kennedy*". It is a great read. Many secrets revealed.
When enough people learn about the OWO and its deeds, things will change. Thus I write this report. There truly is great evil afoot in the world, and we owe it to our country and its founders to learn the truth about it. "Know Your Enemy". Most of us do not.
In Rome's ancient days of glory, The Romans learned how to figure who was doing what by asking the simple question; "Who Benefits?
If the OWO successfully gets Russia and the USA to fight it out with nuclear weapons, who benefits? The USA loses. Russia loses. The OWO wins.

(written in Aug 2022)

Some More Special Bonus Addendum

Pyramid Power
How to shave for almost free!

My dad was an interesting guy. Raised on a farm in Minnesota during the Depression, he didn't have an opportunity to get an education. But he was smart, and had an inquiring mind. He read a lot.

So back in the 1970's he sent me a book titled "Pyramid Power". Interesting book, it elaborated on the special powers of a pyramid built with the geometric ratios of the Great Pyramid of Egypt. In the book, it stated that if you placed a shaving razor at a point 1/3 down from the apex of the pyramid, that the razor would stay sharp.

Many years later, I remembered this. So when I was experimenting with some small replicas of the Great Pyramid, I tried this experiment. It worked. For years I kept my shaving razor sharp with this method. But it was awkward because of the difficulty in keeping a pyramid structure

in the vicinity of my bathroom. The smallest
pyramid that I could fine to use was about 24
inches wide and 19 inches tall. There was never
enough space in my bathroom to use the device.
So I gradually stopped using it.
Here is what I learned: I could use an ordinary
disposable razor. Normally such a razor would
stay sharp for about a week, then had to be
thrown away. I could place it under the apex of
the pyramid. And then it lasted me for up to six
months. Pretty neat. But as I mentioned, it was
very inconvenient to use because of the bulky
size of the pyramid.
Well friends, I have just made another discovery
that I wish to share with you. I have found a very
small brass pyramid that works well to keep my
razor sharp. The brass pyramid is only 2 inches
square, so it fits on my bathroom shelf nicely.
And I bought it on the Internet for less than
$10.00. I placed my razor (shown in the picture)
on the apex of the pyramid as shown. I started
using this disposable razor in January of this
year. It is now August, and the razor is a sharp
as it was on the first day I used it (maybe even
sharper).
Here is a picture of my rig:

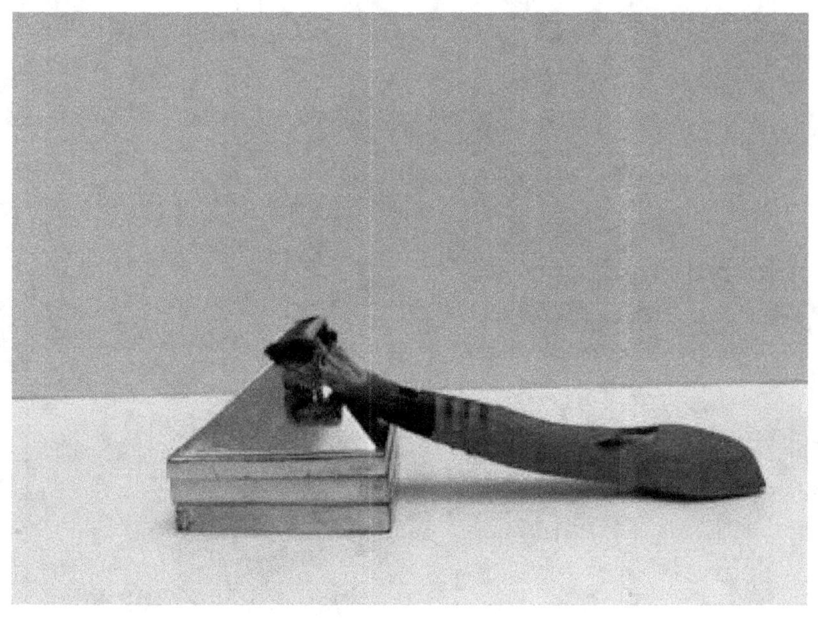

In case any of you wish to experiment with this
rig, you can google "small brass pyramid".
Mine came as a set of 3 pyramids. I stacked
them as shown in the photo for maximum
power.
As I mentioned before, the set of 3 small brass
pyramids cost me around $10.00. Then the razor
cost me about $3.00. If they last for a year, my
total cost of shaving for the year will be $13.00.
Not bad! And I still have the pyramids!
By the way, here is a list of books that I have
written or authored (some with pen names).
They are available on amazon.com.

On Stormy Seas.

Increasing Your Cat's Life & Longevity.

Increasing Your Dog's Longevity.

The Lyme Disease Handbook.

Women's Beauty Secrets.

Defending Against the Ambush.

The Diabetes Handbook.

Salt and Your Health.

Structured Water for Greater Health and Happiness.

Elk Hunting Guide.

Kill Zone.

Egyptian Sacred Geometry.

Pirate History of Florida.

Essiac Story and 6 Examples.

Two Essiac Angels.

Essiac Handbook.

Essiac Testimonials.

A Terrible Beauty.

Sacred Geometry. Healing Water.

Male Menopause.

Greater Longevity. Rediscovering the Philosopher's Stone. Sacred Geometry Pyramid Power	Women's Health Secrets. Beating Arthritis. King Arthur & Camelot

www.ingramcontent.com/pod-product-compliance
Lightning Source LLC
Chambersburg PA
CBHW070657250726
48662CB00001B/161